Preparing for METAMORPHOSIS
Life after the Worst Diagnosis

Kelly Mize

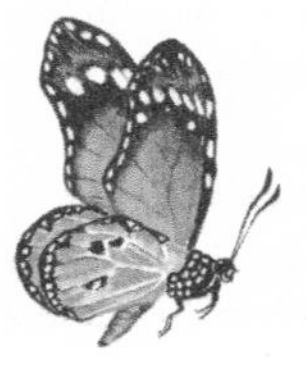

Preface

What is the worst diagnosis? It's the one you've just received. The one that has already begun to reroute your plans, invade your thoughts, and unravel the life you have knit together. My worst diagnosis was terminal cancer, but we are all terminal, all preparing for metamorphosis at some time. The worst diagnosis may escort us to it quickly, as with some cancers and heart conditions, or it may ferry us slowly over years as our bodies deteriorate. Any condition that disables, is progressive, and requires its host to make massive changes to accommodate is a worst diagnosis. Whatever it is, we are living with it ready-or-not, contending with it daily. Because my worst diagnosis ends in death sooner rather than later, that is the perspective I hold.

This book exists only because I have been looking for one that would guide me through the journey I'm on and so far, no such book has surfaced. People who write books on death and dying typically know much about the physiology of death or the spiritual and psychological aspects of it. They are usually medical professionals with knowledge far more comprehensive than mine. These authors are among the robust living, their deaths likely far from imminent. I have read a few of them and found them worthwhile. The book I sought, though, one written by someone living through their last months of life, apparently was living within myself.

I wanted to write that book so that I might better process what is happening to me in these final months of life, and so that others who are in a similar situation might benefit, too. Even if their worst diagnosis doesn't mean imminent death, I hope these chapters still hold something of value as they assess their situation and look for ways to make the most of it. Sharing this story is daunting to me. Awareness of a wider audience than myself changes my approach, and I hereby acknowledge that death from a terminal illness is not a one-size-fits-all adventure. As I contemplate the many ways people make their way through the veil, I realize I cannot speak to all of them. I can only share what has been true for me, and hope that if there are any readers, something in here will resonate with them. My emphasis up front is that I would never presume expertise on anyone else's walk toward their earthly life's closure. To illustrate, let me say who I am, and let the reader decide if it is worthwhile to continue.

I am a fifty-eight-year-old middle-class woman with terminal cancer. My story is told from my point of view as a wife, daughter, mother, grandmother, teacher, and friend. While you, the reader, may not be able to identify with any or all of these roles, you undoubtedly have your own roles and life experiences that parallel mine. We were all living busy lives until illness threw a stick in the spokes, crashing our routines and messing up our plans. The life in which I was immersed prior to my diagnosis was both fulfilling and demanding, and I detail it in my story to set the stage onto which cancer danced, uninvited and threatening to ruin everything.

I was diagnosed with colon cancer in 2017, and through a couple of courses of chemo and radiation, lived several months with no evidence of disease. More recently, the cancer has resurfaced in the form of peritoneal carcinomatosis, which is fatal. I had been a teacher until the spring of 2020, and qualified for disability, so I have a second income consisting of 60% of my former salary. My husband and I have been married thiry-nine years, and he has excellent insurance benefits that have covered my treatments and now hospice care. Many fellow sufferers do not have the safety nets in place that I presently have, and I am sorry. I cannot imagine handling this disease and its decline without my family, without the comfort of my home, and without full insurance benefits as some must endure.

I know of a man whose sister took him in during his last months; he had no home, no insurance, and no one to care for him. She was able to find assistance and arrange hospice for him, thankfully, but prior to her intervention he was suffering alone. Another hard situation is a woman whose son took her in but charged rent during her cancer treatment. While the rent was not outrageous and used to help with household expenses, she had to take a retail job to afford it. She was finally able to get her own place but has had much more to contend with than I've had.

Seeking the camaraderie of fellow patients, I joined a couple of Facebook colon cancer support groups and learned of many people whose spouse or significant other left them because of the challenges of living with cancer. Cancer is distressing for those of us who are patients, but it is also an enormous trial for those closest to us. Their lives are upended too, and some choose not to stay. Desertion is harsh, yet illness does not always bring out the best in us. If we are not mindful that others still have needs, that our personal tragedy isn't the center of the universe, we can exhaust those around us. People are contending with so much more than just the disease. Between relationship crises, demanding employers, uncooperative insurance companies, and tenuous housing situations, the assumption that all readers live in comfort equivalent to mine would be presumptuous. That is someone else's book to write, and without minimizing their suffering, I don't attempt to address those issues here. Besides those genuine difficulties, there are other aspects of terminal illness we all share regardless of financial and social standing.

I am told by my hospice team that those who have a strong spiritual connection seem to fare better as their terrestrial lives end. If that is the case, I will take courage because I am a Christian. This will appeal to some potential readers while excluding others. Acknowledging my faith up front is necessary since it is central to everything I think and believe and write. I do have a child-like faith. My religion is totally a crutch; no, more than that, it is life-support. It is a determination made only after finding other paths led nowhere meaningful, and Christianity is such a rich, joyful way to live that I cannot help but share it. I cannot write anything about my experience without inviting my Lord to be present in each part; He has been present with me throughout everything that has happened, and to exclude Him would be to deprive my writing of its very life source.

Additionally, I'm not dead yet and neither are you. We don't know how we will die even if we have been diagnosed with a terminal illness. There are car accidents, plane crashes, falls, and other potentialities that could beat the disease process to the finish line. Or our disease could end up being an acute rather than chronic situation. For example, cancer patients can have issues with blood clotting, which might cause a deadly stroke or heart attack that cuts short the long, drawn-out disease process. Any of those could happen. As I write, I am operating under the assumption that the long, drawn-out cancer death will be what happens to me, but I acknowledge this may be entirely wrong. I continue anyway, since the probability is high that this is how things will progress.

Preface

The intention of this work is to discuss topics that apply to us all regardless of our financial status, familial support, or spiritual awareness. We all must wrestle internally with our mortality. Even if we are unsure of our spirituality, we must also contend with the notion of what will happen to us when we die, which implies that we are spirit beings. Outside euthanasia, we cannot go over, under, or around it. We can only deal with it daily, and whether that dealing looks more like a dance or a wrestling match depends mostly on our attitudes. When I awaken each morning, the first thing in my awareness is a tangle of thoughts about how to move through the day in the best way possible despite how I physically feel. It takes a minute to breathe, pray, and disentangle myself from any negativity that threatens to ruin the day before it starts. In these pages, I will share the issues with which I strive so that I might live well while dying, then die well in the end. If you, the reader, find yourself in a situation similar to mine, I invite you to join me. I hope you might benefit from my story.

Introduction

This book's structure contains personal reflections that surround a guiding question posed at the beginning of each chapter. I arrived at these questions after four years of journaling about what it is like to live through this experience; they are gleaned from my experiential filter, determining what is most important to consider when we find ourselves at the end of life. The personal reflections, stories, poetry, Scripture references, and interviews all attempt to answer those guiding questions for myself, and I know that each reader would answer them differently. At each chapter's end, I have added ten reflection questions for the reader. I invite you to use the questions to get to the heart of what your experience is teaching you so that you may make decisions with the highest good in mind for yourself and others.

As a former educator, I know that while not everyone enjoys writing, the act of writing helps us sort out our thinking. Speaking does that too, but a written record is helpful so that we may revisit and revise as we go along. Your writing is as private or public as you want it to be. I would encourage using a separate notebook to ponder the questions in writing, though this, like taking medical advice discussed in chapter two, is at your discretion. As my favorite oncologist says, "You're the boss."

Chapter One

Prognostic Awareness

Being realistic isn't the same as giving up.

How can we become comfortable with death?

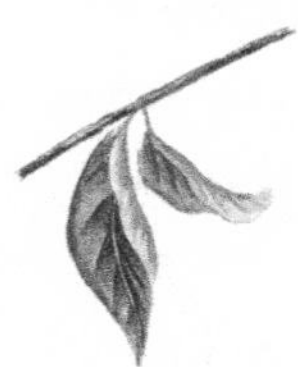

In September of 2009 at 4:00 a.m. our phone jolted us out of blissful slumber and into a jagged, half-conscious awareness that our lives were about to change. It was my mom. "Can you come over? Your dad thinks he's having a stroke." We raced to the closet and dressed, peeling into Mom and Dad's driveway in record time. We entered the house greeted by Dad's attempts to speak. Formerly a man whose deep speaking voice was clear and precise, he was presently only able to utter gibberish. His speech had inflection and nuance, as normal speech would have, but there were no recognizable words. Within minutes, the ambulance arrived, and I rode in the front seat, while my husband, Eric, drove Mom behind us. About halfway there, Dad said, "Kelly, can you hear me? I think I'm okay now. I can talk." I don't remember how I responded to Dad, but my thoughts were troubled. This was no stroke. It had to be something else. He was quickly scanned at the ER, and we had results within an hour of our arrival. There was a sizable mass on his left temporal lobe, and he was to have emergency surgery that day. We all knew what this probably meant, and we were right. The details emerged quickly. The mass was removed, and the diagnosis grim: glioblastoma multiforme, which spreads aggressively and for which there was no cure. Dad accepted the news stoically. We were all in shock, but because Dad himself was such a realist, there was never a moment of denial about what was happening; he was an old pro at understanding his condition and its implications.

Dad had had lung cancer twelve years earlier, treated at M.D. Anderson with surgery and chemotherapy. He knew he might not live, but death was not a certainty, and he wanted to do everything possible to ensure survival. Dad researched and approached his disease with studious, analytical poise. He typed his questions and took the lead role in his treatment, never relinquishing it to the doctors until he was confident in their plans. I was proud of him for being proactive and pragmatic, unlike the many people we have known who passively accept what a doctor says without further investigation. Conversely, he took full charge of his health and ended up cancer-free.

Dad asked his pastor to pray that the Lord's will be done.

This time was different, however. While he was still a pragmatist, there were no proactive measures to take, and so, in Dad fashion, he did what was most reasonable: he asked his pastor to pray that the Lord's will be done. He did not ask for healing, miracles, that it all be found to be a mistake, or any such denial of the facts. He gathered the facts and faced them without flinching. Again, I was proud of my dad for taking this approach, and one of the most important Christian witnesses I have observed was his prayer that the Lord's will be done.

A long-time Sunday sports fan, he seldom attended church for years. I do not know why he eventually acquiesced to my mother's wish (years of fervent prayer) that they could attend church together, but he did. And he did become an outwardly demonstrative man of faith in his attitude and actions, though seldom in words. He became much easier to get along with. Formerly irritable and brooding, and quick to take offense, he became more peaceful, patient, and forgiving. Instead of tense family gatherings where we had to be guarded lest we unwittingly trip a land mine, our times together were much more fun and relaxed. He never discussed or acknowledged the changes that had happened inwardly, but they were obvious and influential. Dad secretly did good works and anonymously paid for people's medications and other needs, never seeking acknowledgement. This is the man my children remember, thankfully. This was Papa, a wonderful grandfather to them, for whom we are all thankful. He loved planning vacations and creating events and gathering people together, so it was fitting that planning a party would be one of his final acts.

When the gravity of Dad's worst diagnosis sank in, he immediately went to work planning a big family celebration for my mom's birthday. He hired catering, reserved the fellowship hall at the church, and put me in charge of the decorations. He made a slide show of their life together to project during the party, then delivered a speech he had written for the occasion, honoring Mom. Nothing in the speech was about him, other than a few remarks about how undeserving he was of such a wonderful wife. He was full of gratitude for her and wanted the world to know it. Once again, I was proud that this man was my father, and his example of humility, love, and courage were profoundly impactful on me, though I did not realize it at the time. These lessons I learned from him, albeit it later in our lives, sank deeply into my own character, continuing to shape my thinking even though I was well into my forties by this time.

Strangely, I grieved his death in advance. We knew his prognosis was bleak, but we did not know how long he had. While Mom was at home caring for Dad, I was working part-time as a consultant, and in November, I went on a training trip to Dallas. While in my hotel room, I had a sudden and overwhelming awareness that Dad would not live much longer. I don't know where this awareness came from, but it was absolute knowledge. I spent that quiet hotel time in tearful acceptance of his impending death. My heart raced, and I sobbed for such a long time, unhindered by distractions at home that would have prevented my processing if I had not taken this timely trip. My arrival back home was met with clarity that his decline was in full swing. I did not tell anyone of my private grief, nor of his death's imminence.

On Christmas Eve, Mom was exhausted and unable to keep Dad comfortable. He had become challenging for her, especially after dark, when he would become disoriented, and she feared for his safety and her ability to manage his care. Mom was his sole caretaker, at his insistence. In his mind, no one else could adequately do the job. Besides her unfailing compassion and devotion, she was his match in terms of being organized. She created a spreadsheet to track medication dosages and frequency, and she deftly handled communication with doctors as he became more confused. Mom's orderly ways astonished the nurses; the small woman in the wheelchair would whip out her annotated spreadsheet when asked about medications, which they photocopied, praising her unusual command of the situation. Despite her weariness, she was smashing it all on her own. While I visited frequently, and my husband and grown children helped with doctor visits and errands, Mom was still the twenty-four/seven nurse aide, helping him with his basic needs. I have no siblings, so I was the only other backup, and though he wanted me to visit frequently, caring for his physical needs was out of the question. Our little family of three had always been modest, and it was a foregone conclusion that modesty would prevail until the end. While Dad and I were comfortable with this arrangement, it left a lot for Mom to handle on her own. For her to concede that she could no longer care for him, I knew the end must surely be near.

Dad's doctor arranged for him to be met at the hospital where he was evaluated and admitted; it was soon determined that he was actively dying, evidenced by mottling on his feet and legs. Within a short time, he was transferred to Harry Hynes Hospice. Mom and I had no idea what blessings were in store for us there, but once the admission process was complete, we were able to rest and let the nurses take over.

The nurses and aides swooped in and immediately attended to the details of Dad's comfort, and they were no less attentive to me and Mom. One nurse gave us booklets describing the physical stages of death after seeing that we were interested in the process, explaining that not all families want to know, and some will not even abide use of the "D" word. We read and discussed the booklets, and I used a computer in an adjacent room to investigate further. While I intuitively had realized this when in Dallas, it was confirmed now that his body had been dying for weeks. What I learned made me wish we had enlisted hospice care long before what turned out to be his last week of life.

Mom had done the work of a team mostly by herself. She could have had nurse aides, a chaplain, a social worker, a nurse—a whole team of people visiting the house and helping with baths, toileting, medications, and spiritual care. We had just not known. Now that Dad was resting comfortably, Mom was able to relax, too, and realize just how hard she had been working. She now had room in her brain to reflect on the past weeks and months and could better understand what she had been witnessing.

Hospice turned out to be such an unexpected treasure. These medical personnel treated him, and us, with such kindness and respect, giving us such comfort and assurance that he was receiving the best possible care. There were nurses who talked to him soothingly, as if he were a small child (yet not condescendingly), those who sang, a chaplain who visited often and offered much wisdom and solace for us, and nurse aides whom God must have made just for the purpose of journeying alongside the dying. I believed this the very day I saw them in action, and my belief was confirmed by my hospice chaplain, Tom. He has worked alongside hospice aides for years and known them to take their work seriously, compassionately caring for fragile, dying bodies in providing their last baths, honored to be entrusted with that role. For him, there are similarities between the last bath and Jesus' last supper with His disciples. The finality in these two acts brings about closure to those most intimate with the dying. For Dad, the aides did their work with such reverence that we began to allow our long-held vigilance to disintegrate, trusting them to carry the load so that we could fully absorb the moments; we now had enough pause to see that there is a certain beauty and sacredness in death just as there is in birth.

Hospice turned out to be such an unexpected treasure.

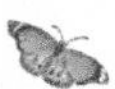

It is my observation that neither of these mysterious events are held as sacred as they perhaps once were, in times when common people were immersed in the full reality of birth and death; such rites were inescapable due to their ordinary occurrence in people's homes. Now, they occur in sterile environments and are left to the professionals. We need not get involved, scrubbing blood and bodily secretions from our hands and our homes, seeing and smelling and touching dead bodies in preparation for burial, or washing waxy, bloody babies before putting them to their mothers' breasts, then attending to placental detritus.

As we have trended toward artifice in these life-affirming rituals, spared the unclean details of attending bodies in all kinds of distress, we have reaped a certain artifice in the rest of our lives as well. The organic details of life have slowly ebbed away over the decades as profit opportunities have made consumer goods and services of them, and it is now possible to live one's entire life without experiencing anything at all the way our ancestors did. Sometimes I get carried away, wishing I had been born in a simpler time and tend to romanticize what life might have been like 150 years ago until I think about how gross those organic details were, or how ibuprofen and Tramadol didn't exist. I'm quite content that the most gruesome medical crises I've ever handled involved bloody noses and Band-Aids. Twenty-first century life isn't all that bad and attending a loved one's death in a hospice setting can be a blessing, where we can be present with them while leaving the physical care to those better equipped. Even better, we can involve hospice care far in advance of life's last days, relieving our relatives of those not-so-romantic details altogether.

As Mom and I kept watch over Dad, the nurses and aides were more intimately connected with his physical deterioration as they kept him clean and comfortable. Despite their work and our desire to accompany him, this was his passage, and we could only go with him so far. Not to overstate the obvious, but this simple thought had never occurred to me: the work of dying (as far as observers can see) must be done alone. As systems shut down and the dying person retreats from the world, the interior work happening in this later stage remains inscrutable to those of us left behind. Medical treatises detail the stages of death and what can be expected at each step within the body, but what about the spirit?

It is far from expiring, but rather emancipating from its worn-out flesh. It is at this juncture that a Christian's hope becomes manifest—more real than our earthly existence ever was. The following Scriptures do not tell us what happens, but they do tell us that we are far from alone.

> Even though I walk through the valley of the shadow of death, I will fear no evil, For you are with me; your rod and your staff, they comfort me." (Psalm 23:4)
>
> Do you not know that you are God's temple and that God's Spirit dwells in you? (1 Corinthians 3:16)
>
> God is love, and whoever abides in love abides in God, and God abides in him. (1 John 4:16b)
>
> No one has ever seen God; if we love one another, God abides in us and His love is perfected in us. (1 John 4:12)
>
> But you have upheld me because of my integrity and set me in your presence forever. (Psalm 41:12)
>
> And behold, I am with you always, to the end of the age. (Matthew 28:20)

The experience common to us all cannot be facilitated by family or friends, but only by God, similar to a caterpillar's conversion to a chrysalis. The caterpillar instinctively finds a suitable branch from which to suspend itself, then hangs for days as its inner recesses dissolve and the transformative work is undertaken. We may observe a chrysalis, or many chrysalides may be suspended together from the same branch, but each one is metamorphosing individually; they cannot help each other. We, the observers, cannot help them. We know that when a butterfly emerges, we are witnessing an intelligently-designed transformation that only a divinely creative Being could manifest. Maybe a spirit's impending departure is something like that as well. The dying retreat deeply into themselves before their hatching, and then in ways we do not fully understand because we cannot see, they are transformed. The Apostle Paul explains our incomplete comprehension this side of the veil, hinting at the full disclosure to come in 1 Corinthians 13:12, "For now we see in a mirror dimly, but then face to face. Now I know in part; then I shall know fully, even as I have been fully known." Further, having placed our faith in Christ, we know these earthly limitations will soon be supplanted by a glorious, revelatory transfiguration. 1 John 3:2 promises, "Beloved, we are God's children now, and what we will be has not yet appeared; but we know that when he appears we shall be like him, because we shall see him as he is."

Before the butterfly escapes its plain, dull chrysalis, it struggles mightily...

These Scriptures comfort and encourage us because we are still bound by our temporal senses. As we witness another's final hours, it is also helpful to remember that before the butterfly escapes its plain, dull chrysalis, it struggles mightily, pushing and tearing the enclosure with all its might before its beauty is revealed and its flight to freedom takes wing.

In Dad's chrysalis phase, he became less communicative over successive hours and days. When he arrived at Harry Hynes, Dad was singing "Mack the Knife," cracking jokes, and asking for a cheeseburger. I learned later that this is a stage in the dying process. People often will rally for a while and behave like their old selves before withdrawing and gradually fading away. As his time trickled away, his ability to speak deteriorated due to the nature of his particular cancer. He could only summon a few words and could not assemble them into collective sentences, but his facial expressions and gestures communicated plainly that he was happy to see people who came to say their goodbyes.

I was especially warmed by Dad's goodbye to his poker friend, Ron, as they shook hands and looked eye to eye. This exchange looked like nonverbal man code as they wordlessly expressed the gratitude for their friendship. When my husband, Eric, came in to see Dad for his final goodbye, Dad worked so hard to form the words "Good guy!" as he pointed at Eric with determined affirmation. He had been pleased to have Eric for his son-in-law, and he communicated it so proudly. His encounter with his granddaughter, Erica, and her son, Gage, were harder for him. There were hugs and goodbyes and tears, then he gazed intently at Gage's tiny features for the last time.

Now the visitations trickled to a stop. Mom and I were his remaining companions, and the real work of dying began to intensify. He slept, or lay quietly much of the time, but there were a few behaviors that frightened us somewhat. I was reading about terminal restlessness as we witnessed it, which helped us understand, but it was startling, nonetheless. He tried to tie the sheets to his bed rails. He sometimes grasped at invisible objects in midair. Absorbed in these fussy matters, he no longer acknowledged our presence, completely secluded inside his agitated physical shell. Once in the middle of the night, he sat straight up in bed, attempting to stand. Mom shielded him while I went for the nurse, who arrived instantly with the calming sedation. And then, he began breathing heavily. His face became increasingly mask-like as the hours passed, not unlike the grim reaper masks we find in stores around Halloween, a disquieting development. The labored breathing, I learned, was called Cheyne-Stokes breathing, which can start and stop for quite a while before ceasing altogether.

Mom and I were quietly visiting at his bedside on the late afternoon of January 1, 2010, while I occasionally scanned the booklet the nurses had provided about the stages of death, and I learned that the last of the five senses to go was the sense of hearing. Wondering if Dad was able to hear us, I walked over to the far side of the bed up by his shoulder. I said,

"Dad, if you can hear me, raise your eyebrows," and he DID IT! We were so stunned to think that he could hear us all along. He seemed to be disengaged from us, but now we saw that we could have been talking to him all this time and hoped he would not think us negligent in just casually chatting all those hours. I told him I loved him, and his eyebrows reached toward his hairline a second time, which I took as reciprocity. Mom spoke some things to him as well, then a few moments later his breathing stopped. Our breathing suspended too as we waited for his next inhalation, but it did not come, and the gravity of the moment struck Mom with a forceful panic. Her heart was racing out of control. I did not tell her this, but I had already had this strange sensation in my hotel room back in November, grieving in advance of the actual death. And then, as her heart rate resumed its normal pace, we stayed with him until the undertaker arrived.

In such a moment, the Scripture verses I shared here do not always come to mind. We thought we were ready, but it's impossible to be ready. Being ready might have included meditating on these verses, but I had not done so. I have often thought of Dad as being with Jesus *in* Heaven, but I had never considered that he was accompanied by Jesus in his passage *to* Heaven until I began to wonder about the one I would soon make.

It was over, for us. Not for Dad. He had been released from his chrysalis and had flown free. This separation was surreal. It could hardly be possible that he had been with us all this time, and now he was gone. We would go back to life as usual, only it wasn't usual at all, especially not for Mom. I would return home to my husband, and our lives would pick up mostly where they left off. Mom, though, was now a brand-new widow.

The account of my father's death ends here but living its reality did not, especially for Mom. Her life was profoundly upended, and it took years for her to find her bearings. Being present to this was difficult because I could not fix it for her. Like Dad enduring his death alone, Mom would have to make her way through grief alone, too. We could accompany her to a point, but we could not go through it with her or for her. While I compared the dying process to a butterfly's development, the metaphor could apply to the grief process as well. A part of Mom's life died, and she had a long period of struggle before she could emerge transformed, functioning fully and feeling alive again.

I describe Dad's illness and death in such detail here because it affected me so significantly. I had never watched another human die. And now, years later and facing my own impending death, I realize that observing others' illness and death affects us indelibly. The way Dad handled his approaching death was seared into my soul, a hidden discovery I made upon receiving my own diagnosis. I have frequently drawn upon his wisdom throughout the past four and a half years and have let his example guide my own decision-making. I hope that somehow, he is aware of how important he is to me, and how influential he still is, especially his last twelve years. The way he handled life and death during those years was his best legacy, and I wish everyone could have such a solid example as mine.

Prognostic awareness is a term used to measure a person's grasp on the reality of their prognosis.

Prognostic awareness is a term used to measure a person's grasp on the reality of their prognosis. It is "the process of understanding your illness . . . and it takes time to develop," according to Vicki Jackson and David Ryan, who wrote *Living With Cancer: A Step by Step Guide for Coping Medically and Emotionally With a Serious Diagnosis.*[1] Much research has been done in identifying factors that influence one's perception of their own mortality, and it is clear to me that Dad saw his situation clearly both times he was diagnosed with cancer. He never denied, engaged in wishful thinking, or sugar-coated the truth. He wanted to live and sought treatment. When the treatment was unsuccessful, he surrendered to the inevitable, but he did not "give up."

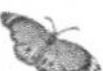

There exists a cultural phenomenon wherein we have created a metaphor surrounding cancer. It is frequently referred to as a battle, both within and outside the medical field. We seem to use this metaphor without realizing we're even doing it. "She lost her battle with cancer . . . " or "He is in a fight for his life" are common expressions, and this easily becomes advice to the cancer patient that sounds like "Don't give up! Fight like hell!" or "You've got this. You're gonna kick cancer's ass!"

These are well-meaning efforts meant to encourage, and often people with cancer use this metaphor themselves. However, there is a downside. When one becomes aware that the treatment is no longer working or is too toxic to tolerate, the metaphor breaks down. It is revealed to have been false bravado all along. What does this metaphor suggest for someone whose treatment is no longer effective? They have lost the battle. What about the person for whom the treatment is too toxic to tolerate? They are weak and have given up. These are defeating and detrimental, and I wish we could reframe the way we talk about cancer.

With my own diagnosis of colon cancer, I never felt like I was in a fight for my life. No battle ensued. Instead, I have sought treatment for a disease, had some good stretches of time without its intrusion, and now that the chemo feels too toxic to continue, I no longer want to subject myself to it. I prayed about this decision because I did not want to make it in haste, nor did I want to base the decision on my chemo-induced physical misery. I wanted the decision to be the right one, and everyone knows that the "right" decision is not always evident until it is seen in retrospect. Because the entire matter was surrendered to God, I have assurance about my decision that I will explain in the next chapter. I have not given up, as has been suggested a time or two by well-meaning friends and acquaintances. There is nothing to give up except a poisonous substance that worked at one time, but no longer offers hope. The treatment has been discontinued. That does not mean I have given up on life, or on wanting to live my life as fully as I can for as long as I can. What it means to me is that I have taken Dad's cues. It's time to recognize the facts and fully face them.

This is prognostic awareness, and it is a healthier frame of mind than denial, or a feeling of having to "keep up the fight" so that we do not look weak to others. I choose to see the situation as clearly as I can and seek the best way to spend the remaining time without trying to maintain a false bravery.

People tell me I am so strong. I know they mean well, and I am thankful for their encouragement, but I am not strong at all; I simply have no other options. I can't very well collapse in despair! Instead, I count among my many blessings two of the resources that substitute for my lack of strength. The first is spiritual provision: daily seeking guidance from the Lord in prayer and in His word, trusting that He will continue to sustain me as he already has many times over. The second is medical support: enlisting hospice early on. Since I am no longer seeking life-extending medical treatment, I want the safety net of medical supervision to monitor and mitigate symptoms as they arise, relieving myself and my family of managing my health on our own.

Your Reflections

1. How have you experienced another's death, and what understanding did you gain through that experience?

2. At what point will you begin to pull away from your doctor's recommendations (if at all) and make your own decisions?

3. What further research might you want to do regarding your options?

4. What has been your own journey to full prognostic awareness?

5. Which aspects of your diagnosis bring you the most grief, and why?

6. Who are your best resources in helping you to get your affairs in order?

7. What are some things you really want to make sure to accomplish (e.g. list valuables and who is to receive them, repairs in your home, attendance at weddings, etc.)?

8. What physical items might make your life more comfortable right now (a new robe, a reclining chair, fuzzy socks, etc.)?

9. What are you putting up with that you'd like to change?

10. *Prayer*: Write out your thoughts, questions, and concerns to God.

Chapter Two

Chemo for Life

Having a doctor you trust is essential, but your own convictions have value, too.

Whose job is it to make decisions about our healthcare?

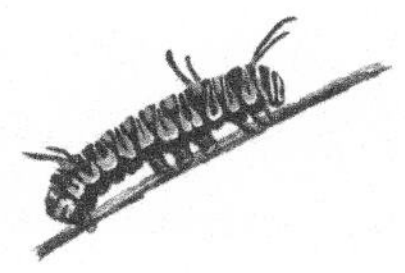

It was the last free Saturday before the 2017-18 school year began: August 10, to be precise. I was sleeping peacefully, dreaming of our back yard. Eric and I have worked as a team over the years to make our back yard a lovely oasis, but in this dream, it was far more: a lush, botanical garden with huge, colorful flowers and shrubs, quaintly winding paths, and immaculately manicured grass and trees. I was marveling at its beauty and reveling in a stroll through its soft, cool grass when I noticed the sunset. It, too, was brilliantly colored with red-orange hues and bursts of golden rays cast upon a halcyon garden I could scarcely believe was ours. This sunset was unusual, though. Where typical sunsets gradually fade from daylight to dusk, this one was setting so rapidly that I panicked, fearing my enjoyment of its serenity might be permanently ending. A last glance around revealed another startling scene: my eye snagged on a corner of the yard previously unnoticed. It was overgrown with thorns and dead shrubbery, thick with unkempt grasses, weeds, and small, gnarly trees. I could see that there was an entrance to it, like a walled garden, but its opening was mostly obscured by untamed, barbed fronds and skeletal branches. How had we managed to keep the yard looking so spectacular without realizing our total neglect of this area? With a growing sense of dread, I saw that there was a flagstone path leading straight to this corner, and I found myself standing on the first stone, knowing I had to walk this path. Upon this realization, a thick blanket of darkness fast enveloped me. Night had fallen swiftly, suffocating every light source with inky blackness. Disappointment grew to vexation as I puzzled over the abrupt nightfall. There was a sense that this garden might represent everything I had ever enjoyed, and that it was coming to a swift, irrevocable end. Overcome by the inescapable conclusion that the corner must be approached, I stood nervously frozen to that first stone until the flagstone in front of it began to shimmer in luminous invitation. I accepted with resignation by stepping onto it, drawing a step closer to the dreaded corner. Riveted to the fading second stone, I was once more cloaked in darkness. Again, the next stone lured me forward, its faint golden glow steadily growing brighter, radiating warmth and light. Obediently, I stepped onto its irresistible platform. Waiting in the quiet stillness, I asked no one in particular, "How are these stones lighting up?" In response, a lantern slowly swept in from my right side, illuminating the next stone. As it gleamed in anticipation of my footfall, an audible voice replied, "My word is a lamp for your feet and a light for your path."

"My word is a lamp for your feet and a light for your path."

Immediately I recognized this from the Psalms, though I could not identify chapter or verse. Also immediate was the knowledge that 1) the hideous corner was an absolute certainty for me, 2) I needed to trust

God, and 3) it would be essential to remain faithful in reading my Bible. That was the end of the dream. I briefly awakened, sleepily registering the remarkable dreamscape that had just played out, returning to a dreamless sleep for the remainder of the night.

Waking several hours later, I descended the stairs in pursuit of coffee, then shuffled to my big brown chair to start the day with the devotional book I had been using, *Jesus Calling* by Sarah Young.[2] It read:

> August 10
> . . . Energy and time are precious, limited entities. Therefore, you need to use them wisely, focusing on what is truly important. As you walk close to Me, saturating your mind with Scripture, I will show you how to spend your time and energy. My word is a lamp to your feet; My Presence is a Light for your path.

Instantly, the dream flooded back into my consciousness; waves of shock and awe engulfed my spirit. The devotional featured Psalm 119:105—the verse spoken in my dream. The odds of having a scriptural dream, then awakening to find the same Scripture prescribed for that day must be infinitesimally small. I had not seen the day's passage in advance. I had not memorized this Scripture. But here it was, spoken to me (by Jesus?) in a dream wherein it appeared. I was about to face something unavoidable and unpleasant, and the best way into it would be to stay immersed in Scripture. I did not know, and still do not, whether this dream had anything to do with what happened a few weeks later, but it seems likely.

The school year began almost normally. Normal for me would have been weeks of enthusiastic brainstorming, list making, and toiling over my classroom's visual appeal, then lesson planning to seize that first week's opportunity to set a positive tone. I was always eager for students to arrive on the first day and couldn't relax until I knew each one by first and last name. I had always wanted to be a teacher, and here I was, living the dream! This year, though, did not come together with my usual fervor.

The usual teacher tasks were accomplished, just barely. I was exhausted for no identifiable reason, and it took every bit of energy I possessed to get the year rolling. My plans were sort of minimally satisfactory, without much creativity. The room looked acceptably neat and organized, but nothing new or creative was added; both the room and the lesson plans lacked inspiration. Nevertheless, the kids arrived, I dutifully taught the lessons, and crashed hard at the end of each day, which every teacher does the first few weeks at the beginning of the year. This time, though, I didn't rebound by mid-September as should be expected. August dragged into September, which slogged into October. Too distracted by school to think much about it, I had dimly registered a pain in my lower left pelvic area for several weeks. I dismissed it, judging it to be an ovarian cyst. Knowing it would resolve in time, I took ibuprofen every four hours and waited it out. Instead of resolving, the pain grew more insistent, so I increased the ibuprofen to the maximum dose. Still, the pain continued.

The first weekend in October, we had planned a camping trip with our daughter and grandsons, and the morning of the trip I was in so much pain that I secluded myself in my office and cried until the ibuprofen took effect. I concealed the pain because I didn't want to cause a canceled trip, disappointing the boys. Pulling myself together, I emerged from my office feeling fragile and uncomfortable but determined. The trip went as planned though I gritted my teeth through most of it, avoiding strenuous activity and snacking on ibuprofen. The kids had fun fishing and hiking, and we enjoyed our evening fires. I hid my misery and worry, but Eric sensed my discomfort and picked up lots of slack that I normally would have handled. I did a lot of sitting around with my sketchbook and didn't really do my fair share of the work, but other than Eric, it seemed to go unnoticed.

And then it was time to return to the classroom for another dispirited week. Starting each morning unrefreshed and exhausted, I trudged through my duties, relieved to go home and collapse at the day's end. Feeling feverish one evening, I took my temperature. Sure enough, it was elevated, and I employed my one and only strategy: ibuprofen. It kept the fever down, enabling me to plod through, finishing the week at last like a collapsing marathoner after mile twenty-six.

Teachers often laugh that they're asleep by 6:00 p.m. on Friday night just as everyone else's party is getting started. On Saturday we have a pulse again, then Sunday we're mobilizing to attack and conquer Monday. On Sunday, October 15, I was not mobilizing to do anything. Something was terribly wrong. The fever spiked again, and ibuprofen proved powerless against both it and the pain. I felt awful all over and called to Eric. "You're gonna have to take me to the ER. Something is really wrong." He wasted no time. On the way there, I called my doctor and described what was happening. "Am I ridiculous to be heading into the ER?" I asked, feeling foolish for being a baby. I needed to get this problem fixed so that I could be ready for work the next day, and I had begun to question myself. Maybe I was making a big deal out of nothing. "No! What you described sounds like diverticulitis, and you definitely need to be in the ER," came his reply. I actually felt better by the time we arrived and had been chatting with the P.A. who was a family friend, and the nurses. This only increased my concern that maybe I was being too dramatic about this nagging little pain.

I employed my one and only strategy: ibuprofen.

The ER doctor came in to report the scan results. He was incredulous at the banter taking place, explaining that when scans look like mine, patients are usually curled up in a fetal position unable to speak. Strangely, I was immensely relieved to learn that I had not been imagining or exaggerating at all. I should have been alarmed, and it seems foolish now, but at the time, it was a relief to know that I had a hole in my colon, justifying all this fuss. The scan showed lots of inflammation due to perforated diverticulitis.

Then he dropped the bomb: I would be traveling to the main hospital via ambulance. He left to make the arrangements, but the P.A. stayed behind and told me that it could rupture, a fatal possibility. Still, I was not alarmed about my health. Looking back, was this shock? Denial? I don't know, but all I could think about was work . . . I had nothing ready for a substitute. I should have been focused on the unfolding situation in my colon, which was evidently leaking its contents into my abdomen, but instead I started texting my principal and coworkers with instructions on what should happen the next day in my classroom since it looked like I might be out for a day or two. A teacher cannot just call in sick without a backup plan, and there are no instructional days to waste so we can't just fill in with pointless time fillers. How had I not anticipated before the weekend that something serious might be emerging? I could have been prepared and saved myself the trouble of explaining the next day's lesson while in the emergency room. Still, I had not grasped the seriousness of the situation.

Then he dropped the bomb.

Arriving at the hospital a short time later, then sending my husband home so he could rest and go to work the next day (I convinced him this was no big deal and there was nothing he could do anyway), I was alone in my hospital bed. I had arrived at shift change, and nurses were busy. No one had been in to provide pain meds yet, other than the Tylenol back at the ER, and all was quiet. My lower abdomen hurt, but I did not care, as a strangely wonderful sensation descended on me. I felt totally blanketed with warmth, peace, and effervescent joy.

I marveled at how I felt no fear and cared nothing about the pain, knowing God was with me. I didn't want this feeling to ever go away. I just lay there basking in His presence, unable to assign words to the glorious feeling. Having very few Bible verses committed to memory, I did know Philippians 4:7 because of a children's song I learned as a Vacation Bible School teacher. Knowing it and experiencing it are worlds apart, though. "And the peace of God, which surpasses all comprehension, will guard your hearts and minds in Christ Jesus" had just become outrageously real. This medical emergency could have prompted any number of emotional responses, but the least likely one would be peace. Yet, I was overflowing with such blissful serenity; it made no sense whatsoever. It surpassed all comprehension. In time, a nurse came in and started an IV then administered Dilaudid, dropping me into a deep, painless, narcotic sleep.

The next morning, Dr. Hayes, a general surgeon assigned to my case by some process only hospital people know, came in and bluntly informed me that I had narrowly avoided having a colostomy bag, and may yet need one. He confirmed the perforated diverticulitis but said that it could also be masking a cancer, and we would not know until a colonoscopy could be performed, though that wouldn't happen just yet since my colon was too fragile. For now, I was on total bowel rest and would be in the hospital all week. This meant communicating a whole week's worth of lessons to a substitute over the phone, which again was my main concern. Once that task was checked, I managed to rest and fully focus on healing without fretting about my classroom.

The colon mended quickly with IV administered antibiotics, and I was released to go home at the end of the week. Oral antibiotics continued, and I resumed teaching for another six weeks until my colon could finally handle a colonoscopy. In my peripheral awareness, I knew the problem might be bigger than what we originally thought. According to Google, there should be no more pain. My family physician confirmed that there should be no more abdominal tenderness, but there was. I could hardly tolerate any pressure on it, which he said wasn't typical. The morning of the colonoscopy, I was wheeled in for the procedure and, it seemed I was awake and in recovery only seconds later. While Propofol does produce that effect, it was also true that I had only been unconscious for about ten minutes because Dr. Hayes was unable to get the scope through the colon. The pictures revealed ugly black swirls of tissue almost closing off the intestine, the contents of which had been moving through an opening about the diameter of a pencil for weeks now. This explained the excruciating pain associated with bowel activity.

Pathology verified that it was indeed cancer.

Eric was left to show the pictures to me and break the news. Dr. Hayes told him that if we approved, he would schedule an operating room because this intestinal mess needed to come out immediately before it ruptured. He gave us the option of waiting but didn't advise it. I opted to get it done, and by 5:00 that evening, was wheeled down a corridor wearing a puffy blue cap and matching snap-up gown. The bed rolled to a stop inside a small vestibule, and our pastor appeared at my bedside. Eric was with me as well, and Pastor Don prayed with us. It was comforting to have him with us, asking God to guide the surgical process. Soon, twelve inches of sigmoid colon was removed, and pathology verified that it was indeed cancer. The concerns about my classroom finally left center stage in my mind as this arresting new development and its implications dawned on me. Finally, my health received full attention.

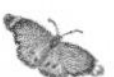

I missed the entire second half of the school year due to surgery, chemotherapy, and radiation. Dr. Zhang, my oncologist, recommended taking a leave of absence if possible, and I was so thankful he did. Many people do continue working throughout their chemotherapy, but I don't know how they do it. Their jobs must be the types where they have a bit more freedom in the workday. Teachers do not have much time for self-care in the school day, and my new condition required much more of it than I was accustomed to. There was no way I could gather the energy to teach classes, grade papers, and deal with the treatment's side effects. Thankfully, I was approved for a leave of absence. Cancer treatment was about to absorb most of my attention, and I was thankful to be able to deal with it unhindered by other obligations.

This first round of treatment would be four rounds of a chemotherapy infusion cocktail consisting of Oxaliplatin, 5FU, and Leukovorin. Together, they are known as Folfox. This was followed by thirty-six daily radiation treatments, ending with four more rounds of Folfox, administered bi-weekly. The treatments were miserable the first week, subsiding after about five or six days. This meant I had a week to recuperate and enjoy feeling mostly normal. Those short reprieves made it possible to continue without becoming too discouraged. It also turned out that I sailed through radiation with very little trouble, for which I was so grateful! The radiation technicians told me this was not typical, as most people do have unpleasant side effects. This time period felt as if it would never end, but it was made tolerable by the kind, compassionate medical personnel I encountered at the Cancer Center and the radiology department at Wesley Medical Center. To a person, each nurse, CNA, doctor, receptionist, and radiology technician were proficient at their jobs and exceptionally caring. I had not a single negative experience and will forever be grateful for them. In total, the treatment regimen went from January to early July, and Eric and I were both elated to have it finished.

Afterward, I healed fast and felt good, and we took a cruise up the east coast to celebrate. I also felt good enough to start the 2018-19 school year with renewed enthusiasm, and even began eating a ketogenic diet, losing about seventy pounds. I hadn't felt this great in years! The school year was a wonderful one, and I enjoyed this class so much. These students had been so much fun, and the school year ended just as well as it had begun. Life had resumed its normal pace, and I began to feel somewhat confident that I had been cured. We enjoyed the following summer with camping trips and yard work and all the activities we usually enjoyed. Life was better than ever. I had experienced a brush with mortality and had given it plenty of consideration, enough to know that every day was to be treasured with humility and gratitude.

School year 2019-20 began with as much joy and anticipation as ever. I had painted my classroom over the summer, adding new furniture and decorations. The room was finally just as I had envisioned. Best of all, I was asked to mentor a student teacher that spring. So far, it looked like this would be my best teaching year yet. After the Christmas holidays, though, I began having trouble with fatigue. I felt depleted, struggling to make it through the day, and a pain gnawed in my lower left pelvic region. Not again. But yes, again. I went in for routine scans, hoping they might reveal anything but cancer, and on February 14, 2021, I went to my oncologist appointment alone. Eric and I had both been in denial that anything could be wrong since I had eaten healthy and felt great for so long. I had convinced myself that scar tissue was responsible for the pain, and the low energy was because it was winter. Isn't everyone low on energy during the winter?

Dr. Zhang reported the disappointing truth: scans and blood work showed the cancer had resurfaced. I had masses on my aorta, left iliac artery, left ureter and ovary, and uterus. Surgery to debulk these masses and perform a hysterectomy would be needed and was scheduled for April. Just as all this news toppled our happy existence, COVID-19 surged across the globe. One might expect that my illness and surgery topped off by COVID-19 would have meant my students received next to no education that spring. Because I had the most extraordinary student teacher, Jordan, the spring semester continued smoothly as she expertly transitioned the kids to online school. I was able to join them soon, and we finished the year successfully. I am still not sure whether Jordan was human or angel. She knew exactly what to do and how to do it, and she truly saved the semester for me and for the students. So, work was managed. Life at home during recovery was another matter.

Her apartment was considered independent living, but the independence ended with the pandemic.

Because of COVID-19 restrictions on nursing homes and assisted living facilities, my mom moved in with us. Her apartment was considered independent living, but the independence ended with the pandemic. Suddenly, her freedom was restricted, so we moved her in with us shortly before my surgery. The bedrooms in our house are all upstairs, and since Mom is a paraplegic, we fixed a makeshift bedroom out of our small library. A room with no door, it provided little privacy. In addition, we had no full bath on the main floor, and she managed hygienic matters with a washcloth and pedestal sink. It was far from ideal for her. For Eric and me, it was a treat. Mom did much of the cooking, which was a blessing. I could recover from surgery without worrying about food. Having her with us did disrupt our routines, but it was also uplifting to have her presence as I adjusted to the fact that I now had stage four colon cancer, drastically reducing my chance of survival. This also meant that I would leave the classroom permanently.

The decision was not easy. I loved everything about my work. The kids, the curriculum, my co-workers . . . I was sad to leave. Eric and I emptied the classroom to make room for someone else to take my place, and I didn't look back. I did not want another year like 2018, where I was in and out, leaving the kids in limbo and having a parade of subs carry the curriculum. It wasn't fair to the students, nor was it easy for anyone involved in making sure the work got done. The teaching chapter of my life had ended, and it was now time to prepare for another course of cancer treatment.

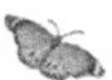

A second line of chemo was prescribed. I was willing to do it to extend life, knowing it would likely not result in a cure. Still, we were optimistic that it might yield several good months. I had gotten seventeen months out of Folfox, and those months were golden. Why not go for another good stint? Treatment began early that summer. It was called Folfieri and consisted of Irinotecan and 5FU, plus a drug called Vectibix, a targeted therapy for my cell type. I spent the summer with a hideous rash on my face and neck, and with debilitating fatigue, but it wasn't too depressing. The side effects were tolerable, and I could spend time outdoors. Just as with the previous chemo, I had a rough week followed by a good one, which made it bearable enough to endure again. There were six rounds of Folfieri. Its side effects were different from Folfox, but I couldn't say one was worse than the other; they were just different but still miserable in their own unique ways. As summer ended, the grand finale of thirty-one radiation treatments ensued. Once again, I breezed through radiation. Dr. Cooke, my radiation oncologist, was so down-to-earth and enjoyable to visit with that I was a little sad to end my time with her. The technicians were friendly and enjoyable as well. The radiation experience, however, has not been missed.

I had gotten seventeen months out of Folfox, and those months were golden. Why not go for another good stint?

Radiation is not painful. As I was radiated, I felt nothing at all. But claustrophobia has long been a little problem for me ever since elementary school. I discovered it on a campout when crawling through a dark, damp cave with my Campfire Girl classmates. There wasn't enough head space to stand in the cave. There were girls ahead of me and girls behind me, and we all had flashlights illuminating occasional spiders. I did not know how far I would be bounded like this and began to panic. Apparently, my freak-out was severe enough that everyone behind me had to crawl back out so that I could escape. This did not win any friendships for me, but I didn't care. Escape was all that mattered! Escape is not an option with radiation. In fact, any movement whatsoever is also not an option. I had to hold perfectly still, the tiny tattoo dots on my abdomen aligning precisely with laser beams. A huge swirling arm circles the bed back and forth at intervals, aiming its invisible rays at the designated target. I learned that the best way to manage the near-claustrophobic treatment was to keep my eyes closed the entire time, reciting the twenty-third Psalm, the Lord's Prayer, bits and pieces of hymns I could remember, and praying for people. Radiation is daily, so I got a lot of praying done. The treatments ended in the autumn.

School year 2020-21 had begun without me, but I was determined to make the best of it and delved into hobbies, church, and enjoying home and family. The treatment did a good job of kicking the cancer can down the road for a while, and I was grateful for more quality time on earth. With so much newfound time on my hands, there was plenty of time for reflection to assimilate what was happening to me, and to our family. Throughout these years of cancer and treatment, I often recalled the dream, believing it to be a caution that I would be going through difficult times, and I took to heart the wisdom of Psalm 119:105. I had been reading my Bible more than ever before and grew in knowledge and understanding. Mostly what I learned was that knowing the Bible is the work of a lifetime, and those who begin young and continue throughout their lives are the wisest among us. My mom is one of these people. Her wisdom has resulted from years of study, demonstrating Psalm 51:6, "Behold, you delight in truth in the inward being, and you teach me wisdom in the secret heart."

She began studying the Bible in her twenties, reading Scripture before going to work. When people say they don't have time to read the Bible, I think of her, rising early to spend time with the Lord, steeping in His word hours before most of us roll out for the day. Her workday ended at 3:00 in the afternoon, when she would come home and make dinner and do her chores, then go to bed early. Our house was always neat and clean, as well. Saturdays were spent doing laundry, ironing, and cleaning while Dad took care of the yard. Those who think it is an imposition to work a full-time job, keep a clean house, and prepare home-cooked meals would be astounded by Mom. She never complained, but it wasn't because she held in her unexpressed resentment. It was because she didn't resent anything at all. She enjoyed her work and did it cheerfully. She never saw housework as drudgery, grateful instead to have a home of her own to manage as she saw fit. Mom had lived a childhood where home was not a safe haven, nor regular meals a given. Cooking and making treats for her family was gratifying, not the joyless grind some would bemoan. Where people who didn't know her saw a sweet little lady in a wheelchair, I knew I was raised by a woman who could beat every man among our family and friends at arm wrestling; their masculinity was no match for her practiced upper-body strength. Her physical strength was matched by her spiritual and emotional strength as well; she had weathered many storms in her young life, applying Ephesians 6:10-18—the armor of God—daily.

> Finally, be strong in the Lord and in the strength of his might. Put on the whole armor of God, that you may be able to stand against the schemes of the devil. For we do not wrestle against flesh and blood, but against the rulers, against the authorities, against the cosmic powers over this present darkness, against the spiritual forces of evil in the heavenly places.
>
> Therefore, take up the whole armor of God, that you may be able to withstand in the evil day, and having done all, to stand firm. Stand therefore, having fastened on the belt of truth, and having put on the breastplate of righteousness, and, as shoes for your feet, having put on the readiness given by the gospel of peace. In all circumstances take up the shield of faith, with which you can extinguish all the flaming darts of the evil one; and take the helmet of salvation, and the sword of the Spirit, which is the word of God, praying at all times in the Spirit, with all prayer and supplication. To that end, keep alert with all perseverance, making supplication for all the saints . . .

Naturally, it could be expected that because of her upright teaching and resilient spirit, I would be a devoted Bible student. I wasn't. We attended a Baptist church in our Wichita neighborhood, where I readily absorbed Sunday School lessons, coming forward in response to the teacher's gospel invitation at eight years old. I understood that I was redeemed by the blood of Christ for my sin by believing in Him and trusting Him to guide me and was soon baptized by immersion. For a time as a fourth grader, I took my brand-new King James Bible to school to read during recess, but it was mostly incomprehensible, and I eventually gave up. Because we had moved into a country rental house several miles from church, our attendance trickled to a stop. Mom and I wanted to continue, but Dad did not, for reasons I never knew other than the twenty-minute drive it took to get there. On the dwindling Sundays we did go, the mood in the car was strained. Dad made it clear that he was going under duress, and Mom backed off. After dropping out altogether, Mom was my only source and example of Christian education. She continued her efforts into my teens, but likely saw little result.

The seeds she planted grew into spindly, delicate sprouts that hung on tenuously for several years, even dormant at times.

The seeds she planted grew into spindly, delicate sprouts that hung on tenuously for several years, even dormant at times. Throughout my adult life, growth occurred sporadically then more steadily as I matured into my forties and fifties. Now, cancer has removed all competing interests. Regret over my slow, decades-long growth is wasted energy, but I know that my limited lifespan will curtail what could have been a much deeper knowledge. One lifetime is scarcely enough to fully comprehend every nuance in God's word. Still, my faith deepened, and my dependence on Christ intensified as my sense of mortality became real and immediate, no longer an abstraction for some distant future date. So, I was late to the party, but I'm here now. I don't know as much as many Christians, but I'm working on it. I look in the mirror and find much inadequacy, but thankfully God has no limitations, and He works with us in whatever condition we arrive at the cross. As 1 Timothy 1:15 assures, "Christ Jesus came into the world to save sinners . . . "

Trusting God became a matter of life support...not just ritual or habit.

While I do not know as much as I feel I should at this late hour, I am content to be known by the One who knows all. 1 Corinthians 8:2-3 reassures me: "If anyone imagines that he knows something, he does not yet know as he ought to know. But if anyone loves God, he is known by God."

Having established new routines for Bible reading and prayer journaling as a result of this newfound free time, trusting in God became a matter of life support as I mentioned in the introduction, not just ritual or habit. The old hymn, "Turn Your Eyes Upon Jesus," became real to me as I resonated so much with the phrase, " . . . and the things of earth will grow strangely dim, in the light of His glory and grace." Immersion in God's word had become far more interesting to me than any fictional plot in a novel or any five-star movie.

There came a time when my entire perspective on life shifted, and I wondered how I could ever continue feigning interest in the amusements that seem to be of great interest to many. I did not consider myself holier or better than anyone else, because I knew I had been just like them before my cancer diagnosis. Cancer escorted me to this contemplative state. There is total peace and complete freedom in this place, even though it came at a cost. For these reasons, I can give thanks for this disease that has otherwise been unwelcome. Is this what it took to make me stop and pay attention? If so, then so be it. The Apostle John explained this centuries ago in 1 John 2:17, "And the world is passing away along with its desires, but whoever does the will of God abides forever."

This peace also gives me a better understanding of James 4:13-14,

> Come now, you who say, "Today or tomorrow we will go into such and such a town and spend a year there and trade and make a profit"—yet you do not know what tomorrow will bring. What is your life? For you are a mist that appears for a little time and then vanishes.

Older people are often heard to remark on the swift passage of time, how quickly children grow, or how some event seems as if it happened yesterday. As I have grown older myself, I get this. In a recent visit with my son Logan, I was that older person lamenting time's flight, but he, in his late thirties, seemed to have a keener sense of it than I did. He believed the problem wasn't that it flies quickly, but that time is deceptive. He was right and both of us knew it, but neither could explain the deception itself. Perhaps the mystery is not that time is vanishing; it is we who are vanishing. We are the mist that appears for a little while, says James. We are a vapor.

The notion of life as a vapor hangs like Florida air in July before me, now that my life has months or weeks remaining. I can see and feel it, but it cannot be fully grasped. Instead of panic, though, I have peace provided by the advice taken from my dream. "My word is a lamp for your feet and a light for your path." That advice, spoken in first person, comes from this actual wording: "Your word is a lamp to my feet and a light to my path." The psalmist declares it in his prayer to the Lord. In his own story, in his own time, he walked the same path we all must walk, and God's word gives us clarity, comfort, and rest as we traverse it.

In my story, the next stone appeared.

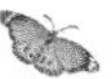

By the time March of 2021 arrived, I had spent several months enjoying life without cancer's intrusion, but I had developed some pretty comical issues with a hernia. It made itself known at such inconvenient and hilarious times, but the worst was when my cat escaped the house late one rainy night. I rushed out to the Tahoe, heedless of the fact that I was barefoot and wearing a thin, white nightgown. I drove around the block and spotted the cat under a nearby vehicle. Slamming my own into park right in the middle of the street, I jumped out onto the wet pavement to fetch him. My lurching Sasquatch moves were no match for his feline stealth. He darted out into the street, deftly eluding my ungainly clutches and flitted under the Tahoe, which meant that I was now trapped, desperately pleading with all three members of the Trinity to divert all traffic since I was blocking the street as well as being completely drenched in my now-translucent gown. I scrambled on the wet, knee-shredding asphalt, my blundering swipes useless against his furtive kitty maneuvers.

Complicating the rescue effort, my intestines had some moves of their own, gushing repeatedly through the fragile hernia over and over. I would jump up, stretching my arms overhead to coax the unruly bowel back in place, then get down and wallow in the street again until at last I managed to grasp his tail and reel him in. After ten minutes of old cat lady in a wet nightgown leaping awkwardly around her car in the rain, the cat rescue mission was accomplished! Because there were no viral videos of the escapade, I trust there were no observers to record it, but once assured of that, my attention was turned to this annoying hernia.

I finally made an appointment for a surgical consult to get it repaired before it could make a repeat performance.

The surgery took place in May, and I asked Dr. Hayes if he would scout around in my abdomen and remove anything lurking that shouldn't be in there. Following the surgery, he reported to Eric that he did remove a spot near my bladder, bustling away to his next patient before Eric could formulate a question. The following week, Dr. Zhang elaborated, telling us that we were now dealing with peritoneal carcinomatosis, a fatal condition. It resulted from the perforation in 2017, and we always knew this was a possibility. Those cancer cells leaked through the intestine into my peritoneal cavity, where they were free to set up shop wherever they liked. This was bad news, but we agreed that since I felt good, I should continue living normally until symptoms arose. I made it until January of 2022 before having any real trouble.

Although I did have mild abdominal pain, it was easily controlled by a ureter stent (to prevent the ureter from kinking) and low dose Tramadol. These simple measures served well until we had just returned from a family trip to Nashville. A couple of nights later, I began to feel considerably worse, mainly with vomiting and fatigue. As it happened, my appointment with Dr. Zhang was already scheduled. He told me that I was experiencing disease progression and would need chemo to push the cancer back. Four treatments of Folfieri plus Vectibix again were prescribed. I felt terrible on the day of the appointment and a little panicked at the idea of receiving treatment already, but we moved ahead anyway.

Treatment began immediately after the appointment, and I discovered that I was woefully unprepared. Where this treatment had been tolerable months before, it felt incredibly toxic now. I was barely able to control the nausea, had uncontrollable diarrhea, became dehydrated, and was in total misery. The fatigue was so debilitating that I felt nearly unable to take care of myself. Getting to the bathroom, brushing my teeth, or taking a shower were overwhelmingly taxing. I remember looking at a basket of laundry that needed putting away, longing to be able to do it so that I would have clean underwear and socks in my drawer without searching, but I was afflicted with such mental and physical torpor that such a demanding chore could not be performed.

In addition, I was constantly cold and could not get warm, thirsty but unable to tolerate drinking, repulsed by smells by which I was continually surrounded such as hand soap or deodorant. In the prior rounds of this treatment, I could expect five or six days of discomfort, which was tolerable because an end was in sight. This time it was misery that took two full weeks to abate, and another week to gradually recover some sense of normalcy.

The treatment was scheduled for every twenty-one days instead of fourteen as originally planned, thankfully. I had barely begun to feel human again when it was time for my second treatment. We met with Dr. Zhang beforehand. What he told us was incredibly distressing, given my response to the Folfieri/Vectibix brew. He said I would need to continue treatment until it became too toxic or until the cancer grew despite it.

In other words, chemo for life. I floated down the corridor, dazed, for the second treatment with these words swirling through my soul . . . chemo for life. Eric was with me, and I knew he was brooding over it too. This was not what we had understood previously. We believed there would be four treatments, then a break until symptoms arose again. Dr. Zhang had not deceived us. Rather, he wisely dispensed just enough information at each visit so that we only dealt with the situation at hand. It would

In other words, chemo for life.

be impossible for him to foretell everything that could possibly happen, and unfair for us to expect him to make those predictions. If I had it to do all over again, he is the oncologist I would choose, and I am so thankful for him. Still, this was the day he had to deliver the sour news: chemo for life. Both of us were quiet as the nurse came in to connect my port once again to the poisonous drip. I had not seen it that way previously, but this time that was all I could envision . . . my unwilling body infused with the toxic cocktail that would bring another episode of wretched misery. It was made better by my daughter, Erica, who committed as she had done before to take me for IV fluids two days after the chemo drip, but still, it wasn't enough to relieve the sensation that I had eaten a box of rat poison.

This treatment was just as hard as the first had been, and after several days of unrelenting misery, I realized there would be no way to reconcile with "chemo for life." There was simply no way my body was going to put up with it one more time, let alone for the rest of my shortened life. I prayed but had no discernible guidance from God other than the feeling of utter dissonance and inner conflict at the prospect of continuing. I have found that although guidance doesn't always come instantly, seeking God first before major decisions is always advisable. 1 Peter 5:6 instructs: "Humble yourselves, therefore, under the mighty hand of God so that at the proper time he may exalt you, casting all your anxieties on him, because he cares for you." Even as I did this, my instincts screamed that there was no point in more chemo, no quality of life at all under its influence. The very thought of enduring treatment repeatedly was agonizing, which made the decision to stop treatment an easy one.

Once the decision was made, I felt immediate relief despite knowing the prognosis would be shorter. I physically felt lighter, even breathing more easily. After telling Eric, who understood my predicament because he had been in such anguish (his word choice) watching me suffer, I called the Cancer Center and canceled the next treatment. My next call was to Phoenix Hospice to schedule a visit with a hospice nurse and friend, Beth. A couple of days later, the third call was to the Cancer Center again, requesting that Dr. Zhang write an order for hospice. Within a few days, the admission process was done, and the relief was so refreshing. Taking the matter to God, then making these proactive moves rather than passively accepting chemo for life lifted my sense of despair. I recognized that I did not have to consent to anything that gave me that much trepidation, and I credit my dad for this, too. His example showed me that I was free to make decisions about my healthcare, something that seems unrecognized by many people. Every trip to the Cancer Center I see people who are wheelchair-bound, too weak and exhausted to stand or walk. Their skin is gray, their eyes dull, and they look miserable, but they have come to the Cancer Center for another chemo infusion in hopes of squeezing a few more days of life out of the calendar. This is their choice to make, and I respect it. I just hope they have made the choice rather than defaulting to their doctors' counsel. I always told myself that if I reached the point where treatment no longer offered hope of good extended time, I was done. The decision would be mine to make.

Taking the matter to God, then making these proactive moves rather than passively accepting chemo for life lifted my sense of despair.

Remembering Dad's first encounter with lung cancer demonstrated the importance of taking responsibility for one's own health. He had gone to an oncologist who told him he had stage four lung cancer and should get his affairs in order. I was with Dad at this appointment, and this doctor seemed completely certain of his judgment. Dad went home in sadness and resignation, but these soon transformed into determined analysis. He began to research and study his cancer type and learned that some of the diagnostic tests typically used in his situation had not been performed. His doctor had made his diagnosis based on incomplete information. What he did know was that there were two masses on one lung, enlarged lymph nodes in the mediastinum (which the doctor said meant the cancer was transferring to the other lung), and nodules on the liver. He typed a long list of questions based on his pathology report and other items he had found in his investigation.

The response was not positive. "It doesn't matter what tests we do; you're going to get the same result." Dad said he wanted copies of all his medical records, and that he wanted to go to M.D. Anderson in Houston. The doctor was immediately defensive and told Dad it wouldn't make any difference. Undaunted, it was clear to Dad that this condescending doctor was overconfident. We were soon on our way to Houston. All the recommended diagnostics were performed, and the results were gratifying. There was no cancer in the mediastinum; even though the lymph nodes were enlarged, it turned out Dad was a person who had large lymph nodes everywhere, so these were not exceptional. The liver nodules were benign as well. This meant that Dad had stage two, not stage four, and his cancer was entirely curable. He had a pneumonectomy and several treatments of Carboplatin and Cisplatin, and for twelve more years he was cancer-free.

Knowing one's own condition and taking responsibility for medical care decisions is essential for best results.

We learned from this experience that to have total faith in a doctor is naïve. Knowing one's own condition and taking responsibility for medical care decisions is essential for best results. We, the patients, are in the driver's seat. Respecting a doctor's professional expertise is good. Surrendering one's mind and will out of obedient deference, passively accepting whatever treatments are offered, is not.

Dad's lung cancer treatment at M.D. Anderson took place in the late nineties, and much has advanced since then. One of the appealing features of this cancer center was the team approach to patient care. Doctors met and consulted on each case, presenting opinions and recommendations for patient consent. Two decades later, this is standard practice in other cancer centers, too, and as I understand it, Cancer Center of Kansas uses this approach as well. They have what is called Tumor Board, where cases are presented for consultation with colleagues, then recommendations are presented to the patient. Now that I was the cancer patient, I was reasonably confident in Dr. Zhang and his treatment plan, knowing my case had been reviewed by a team of professionals at Tumor Board. I gave consent to everything he recommended until these last two treatments, which forced me to realize that it was time to make my own decisions. We weren't talking about saving my life or even prolonging it much. We were talking about disease management through continuous chemotherapy. This was where my confidence in his recommendations ended. He had been an excellent doctor and I continue to be grateful for his work on my behalf, but it was time for me to relieve him of the responsibility for my health. I decided that blasting my weary body with more toxicity was not the answer. It was time to consult with hospice.

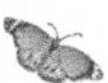

My first meeting with Beth, my hospice nurse, was a comforting relief. She explained how home hospice would work, and all the ways they are able to manage pain and suffering. They also offer chaplain and social worker services in addition to nurse aide help for hygiene care toward the end as needed. She told me that while I am still feeling good, she would come twice weekly to monitor, manage medications, and record my vitals. It was important to me to have this safety net, a team of people who would be supervising my decline and helping me manage it. This also brought Eric and me a sense of calm. Something Beth explained, while still maintaining respect for my doctor, was that people in the medical field are trained to do everything they can to preserve and protect life. This is their orientation to patient care, and when patients are in decline, even drastic decline, they are hesitant to end life-preserving care. Part of this might be because patients and their families expect to be given hope and don't want to hear that death is imminent, and part of it is the desire to do everything possible to save patients. While this is admirable and understandable, one last look at Dad's case reveals just such a futile case in point.

Soon after Dad was admitted to the hospital on Christmas Eve with his progressing brain tumor, a nurse aide gave him a bed bath during which he had a mild heart attack. He didn't know he was having one, but his heart monitor alerted the nurses, and they rushed into the room to check on him. An ultrasound revealed that he had a blood clot from his ankle to his groin, a cancer-related complication. The blood clot had precipitated the heart attack, and Dad's oncologist arrived with a plan. We were incredulous at what this plan entailed. He recommended an umbrella stent be placed in Dad's groin to prevent further heart attack or stroke. Dad said, "Is this an attempt to prolong my life?" The doctor replied that it was the best he could do, and yes, it might give him some more time. Dad said he couldn't think of a better way to go than to have a massive heart attack or stroke rather than prolonging his life with brain cancer. The doctor apologized that he couldn't do more, which Dad understood, holding him blameless. Within a half-hour of his departure, a nurse pointed out the mottling on Dad's feet and legs, a sign his body was shutting down. If he had agreed to this surgery, it would have taken place just days before his death.

Where the first oncologist had been quick to pronounce a death sentence, this one wanted to provide a life-prolonging measure knowing Dad was at the end. I say this not to malign doctors. They are doing what patients and families expect of them: preserving life as long as possible. It is possible that a doctor might never recommend hospice at all, even when it is obvious that life is ending. Hospice, on the other hand, is about helping patients live well while dying. They do nothing to prevent death, and they do everything to make sure patients are comfortable and as pain-free as possible, even well in advance of the end. It is essential for those of us at the end of life to understand these fundamental differences. Fully understanding the difference in orientation can mean that a terminally ill patient and his family might have a better sense of when to make the shift from one type of medical service to the other.

Hospice, on the other hand, is about helping patients live well while dying.

I am presently in the early stages of my hospice experience, and so far, it has been a good decision. Earlier in the year I joined a couple of Facebook colon cancer groups, and every day I read about cancer patients who are in similar situations to mine. Most of them think they must continue chemo, and the commenters almost always tell them to keep fighting. Some of them advise a second opinion or recommend a well-known clinic. A few of them, though, recognize that it is time. There comes a time. Everyone has a time, sooner or later. Facing this and dealing with it work far better than denying and hoping for a miracle, or assuming we are required to continue treatments. There are no requirements and no rules. We must determine for ourselves when it is time to call off treatment, a decision best made prayerfully. We must accept mortality, and surprisingly, acceptance is freeing. Perhaps I say this because I know what lies beyond my acceptance of mortality. God has provided the light for my path with His word. My confidence is in Him and in the life to come, not in endless medical intervention and vain efforts to prolong the inevitable.

Having an acute sense of one's mortality may drive us to do things we would not ordinarily do. In my case, I experimented with poetry as a way of expressing things I couldn't figure out how else to say. I wrote this sonnet on February 8, 2020. It is a reflection on the dream's application, and subsequent prayers that whatever happened would bring about good.

Second Chance

A gracious invitation in a dream—
To read the words of life the Spirit wrought.
Then falling, ill and death-bound so it seemed,
Rebounded; given life another shot.
So suffocated in the day to day
Inertly down below the surface, still;
The dedications earnestly were prayed
Now trampled underneath a wearied will.
To resurrect those once so fervent prayers,
I ask that I may serve as You've designed
To pass the everlasting Source; to share
With hardened hearts the quiet peace of mind.
Restore, refresh, renew, and bring about
Your plans for your beloved and conquer doubt.

Your Reflections

1. What is the story of your health, and how has it led to the current status?

2. To what extent do you have peace with your doctor's treatment plan?

3. What are some things you have done or would like to do to take charge of your health care decisions?

4. What is your greatest healthcare concern right now?

5. What kind of care would feel most comforting to you when you know your time is ending?

6. What might be the best location for you to spend the last days and weeks of your life?

7. How might you like your surroundings to be at the end (quiet, music, Scripture reading, family talking, etc.)?

8. What misgivings might you have about hospice care?

9. What challenges are you facing regarding making final decisions?

10. *Prayer*: Write to God about your worries and concerns, and ask for His guidance.

Chapter Three

Fear of Suffering

Death isn't the problem—pain and suffering are.

How can we face hard things without living in terror?

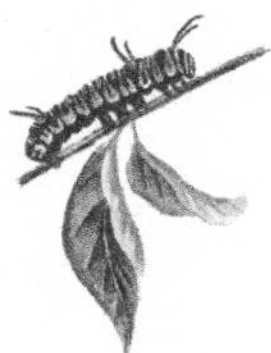

I am tied to the train track, listening for the whistle. Powerless to escape, I know the whistle will eventually sound, signaling the oncoming train by which I will be obliterated. I had been thinking about my situation in this way lately, and I found that it caused me to feel heavy and inert, as if nothing I could do would matter at all. This thinking is recent. Prior to January 2022, I was living with cancer successfully. While it influenced my daily life in terms of energy level and strength, I was able to live normally without thinking about it much. I knew I was terminal, but the actual end was somewhere in the distant future. The visit to my oncologist and subsequent chemo treatments have removed my illusion of the future being distant, and my decision to terminate treatment brought a finality I hadn't sensed until now. What I knew to be true all along is now becoming real, and I am daily discovering how to live with it.

Considering that this phase could still probably go on for months, I realized I could not continue to live with the train metaphor. What a debilitating thing to wake up to each morning: defeat and despair. During those last two chemo treatments, it was easy to feel defeat because of the physical suffering; there is a direct connection between one's physical and emotional state of being. The work of moving through a day, no matter how we feel, begins in our hearts. First, I must realize I do not want to let despair govern the day, and second, I must make my attitude transcend these circumstances. No way can I accomplish that. Therefore, I must appeal to the One who can, which means the answer is to begin the day with prayer.

These kinds of prayers, at least for me, are desperate. When I feel rotten, I have no deep thoughts, and none directed toward the needs of anyone else, at first. I'm thinking of my own abysmal self. How am I ever going to get my teeth brushed? What can I wear that looks like clothes but feels like pajamas? How am I going to make it downstairs to take my meds? All about me, me, me. No Scripture comes to mind, either. I'm too addled for that. I just pray a desperate prayer that sounds something like, "Jesus, help me." I might say it several times in a row. And He always does. Later, when the day is going much better, I open my Bible to find encouragement like this in Psalm 90:14, "Satisfy us in the morning with your loyal love, that we might sing for joy and be glad all our days." When my misery has been brought under control, I can then remember I'm not the only person on the planet and begin to pray for or reach out to others. I find solace in verses like 2 Corinthians 1:4,

> Who comforts us in all our affliction, so that we may be able to comfort those who are in any affliction, with the comfort with which we ourselves are comforted by God.

Oh yes, other people are having a hard time too. Taking my eyes off myself continues to improve my attitude, and He keeps helping in this way, all day long.

The "Jesus, help me" prayer is attached to an especially humbling story from a few years ago. I was working a booth at a medical convention and was feeling especially put-together and professional that day. Feeling elegant in my simple outfit of black slacks and a white blouse accented with tasteful jewelry, my pleasure in my appearance was further enhanced by having an excellent hair day. Everyone at this medical convention was dressed impeccably, and my ego blazed brightly, knowing I fit right in. To everyone's quiet horror, one woman mingling clumsily throughout the room did not. She wore a bright yellow, spaghetti strap shirt, cut-off jean shorts, flip-flops, and had numerous tattoos. Her hair was clean and combed, but was a harsh, brassy gold, not unlike her nicotine-stained teeth. She walked up to my booth to inquire of the weight-loss product I represented, admitting that she needed to lose thirty or forty (I figured sixty) pounds, but that she was concentrating for now on just quitting smoking. "One big change at a time!" she laughed.

She had just schooled me hard.

Feeling slim and superior, I gathered literature and samples for her as she chatted. Her husband was one of the doctors (poor guy) here, and she had come along for the ride. I asked her how she was doing with her smoking cessation efforts, and she said it was tough. Some days, she knew she had no strength to resist the addiction at all. Then she threw a brick at my head by saying, "I just pray 'Jesus, help me.'" She explained her feeling of powerlessness against the long-held addiction, but that Jesus helped her every time. She smiled her sincere, golden smile at me and turned away. Having popped my billowing ego like a pin on a party balloon, she had just schooled me hard. I have never forgotten her simple prayer or her humble witness, unafraid to proclaim Jesus to a total stranger—even one so well-dressed and overconfident. She did indeed stand out in that room full of white enamel and sleek coiffure—her faith in Christ set her apart, and I have no doubt that the Father was well-pleased in His brassy-haired, tattooed servant that day, unlike His fit, fashionable one. At that time, I had little experience with suffering, and could not imagine the desperation that might lead to such a visceral prayer. That is embarrassing to admit. In my soft life, I have experienced some hard times in which a prayer like that might have been a good thing, but I hadn't thought to do it. My encounter with this saint has been pivotal. I now know what it is to have an acute knowledge of my need for Christ, and to have nothing but impatient, intense, primal pleading. Because of her, I know that in those moments, "Jesus, help me" is enough.

Thankfully, those moments have not occurred often. Usually I just feel a dull pain. It's in that same lower left pelvic area and low back. People who aren't terminal could have a pain like this, pop a Tylenol, and assume they'd done something to strain a muscle (or maybe think of it as an ovarian cyst . . .). Those in my condition could, if we let ourselves, hop on the worry-go-round. Is this advancing disease? Is the cancer wrapping around my vertebrae? Will I need to increase my pain med dosage? What if it keeps progressing and tomorrow it's worse, which means I'm soon to be entirely debilitated? What if this means the end is sooner than I thought?

These worries might be legitimate and could easily be true. The real question is, so what? What if I knew for certain the answers to these questions? Did I think I would be in a holding pattern forever, enjoying each day into infinity? So, it could be that this pain I'm feeling is cancer related. Okay then, how does that impact right now, and what can I do about it? Besides remembering to mention it to Beth, who might adjust my pain meds, it means nothing today. While the pain could be a harbinger that something is developing and will increase in discomfort, no physical action can be taken against it.

These are "Oh yeah, I'm on hospice" moments. I sometimes forget I'm on hospice, and the goal isn't to make things go away, the goal is to be comfortable. We are past the "make things go away" point, since we know that isn't going to happen. But what to do about those nagging thoughts, especially the ones that start with "what if"? Those are the most pointless.

Again, I can apply what I know from Scripture to suffocate those intrusive, troublesome thoughts. Remembering Paul's admonition in 2 Corinthians 2:10 to take every thought captive, obedient to Christ, I recognize an opportunity here to apply his words. These fearful thoughts and negative emotions do not come from Him, and I reject them. Instead, 2 Timothy 1:7 says that "God gave us a spirit not of fear but of power and love and self-control." I can take control and choose which thoughts will get the most attention, then meditate on these verses that return me to serenity. Terror of the train loses its grip. When I remember this, to surrender the thought to the One who can discard it for me and replace it with something more productive, I am released from dreadful and foreboding thoughts. It has been interesting to note the means by which they dissipate. They don't always just vanish. A number of things might happen to chase them away. Sometimes a friend or family member will call or text with an encouraging word. At other times, it is a passage in a book that gets my attention or writing in my journal will dispel anxiety. It never happens that I just get stuck in this place of despair.

> **These fearful and negative emotions do not come from Him, and I reject them.**

Another Scripture for which I am so thankful is Psalm 46, where I read that we have a refuge and strength, an ever-present help in trouble. I need a refuge. I am weak and need strength. He is there to provide it and is truly ever-present. The breathless feeling of approaching doom is revealed as a mere phantom, a tactic of my enemy. Why should I fear? We are only here for a little while anyway. Psalm 39:4 reminds, "O Lord, make me know my end and what is the measure of my days; let me know how fleeting I am!

The world offers a full menu of positive platitudes, self-help books abound, and social media keeps us amply supplied with memes to counter negative thinking, but none seem to apply to that strange anteroom between learning of one's impending death and the actual event. I read about one cancer patient who used escapism to occupy her mind by binge watching several Netflix series. I suppose this could do the trick for a while, but those fears will rush in the minute the TV is off, and I need something with more power to carry my mind and spirit to a better place than Netflix. I have found that there is no television show, no novel, and no habit or hobby that can remove the awareness of my condition that continually flickers on the screen in the back of my mind. It's often not dreary and dark, but it is ever-present.

We can't compare our suffering.

A friend who lost her young adult son in a tragic accident once told me she could sleep reasonably well at night, but the moment she awakened each morning, the awareness of her loss nagged unrelentingly during every waking hour until she returned to sleep. Another friend shared that her small son, who had died in her arms of an illness long ago, still sometimes wakes up screaming. We can't compare our suffering. There is always someone whose experience is worse. I don't think my experience compares to theirs; losing a child would be far worse for me than losing my own life. But I understand the sensation of having that constant reminder, and how it can become a burdensome intrusion. In seeking relief from the cumbersome mental and emotional load, I made an accidental discovery.

Reliance on familiar Scripture and taking every thought captive are helpful, but there is something else I found out by accident: reading anyplace in Scripture eliminates fear-based, dread-filled thinking. This is counterintuitive because the Bible cannot be found in the self-help section at Barnes and Noble. Neither is it stocked in the psychology section. Nowhere in the Bible am I going to read about someone suffering from terminal cancer. I'm not going to find a set of instructions for how to handle the last months of life. So, on first examination, I have no explanation for why reading it makes me feel better. Sometimes I can be reading it half-aware of what it's even saying, and I realize I'm in over my head and don't know enough to comprehend a passage or chapter. It doesn't matter. When I've finished reading it, I simply feel better. Yes, I just said I sometimes read the Bible without understanding it, and it still makes me feel better. That doesn't make any sense at all. I asked Eric about this to see if it was true for him too. In customary Eric fashion, he thought about this carefully before responding. Then, he aptly summarized it. Reading Scripture makes him feel more settled. What a perfect word to capture the effect of immersing one's mind in Scripture. When our thoughts and emotions are stirred and we feel disturbed, God's word settles us. The Oxford English Dictionary defines "settle" as to make calm or quiet, and that's just what it does. What does God's word say about itself?

> Do not be conformed to the world but be transformed by the renewal of your mind, that by testing you may discern what is the will of God, what is good and acceptable and perfect. (Romans 12:2)

> The word of God is living and active, sharper than any two-edged sword, piercing to the division of soul and of spirit, of joints and

> of marrow, and discerning the thoughts and intentions of the heart. (Hebrews 4:12)
>
> All Scripture is God-breathed and is useful for teaching, rebuking, correcting and training in righteousness, so that the servant of God may be thoroughly equipped for every good work. (2 Timothy 3:16-17)
>
> The grass withers, the flower fades, but the word of our God will stand forever. (Isaiah 40:8)
>
> Heaven and earth will pass away, but my words will not pass away. (Matthew 24:35)
>
> The unfolding of your words gives light; it imparts understanding to the simple. (Psalm 119:130)
>
> In the beginning was the Word, and the Word was with God, and the Word was God. (John 1:1)
>
> Whoever believes in me, as the Scripture has said, "Out of his heart will flow rivers of living water." (John 7:38)
>
> For the word of the Lord is upright, and all his work is done in faithfulness. (Psalm 33:4)

What message was given to me, personally, in that August 10, 2017 dream?

> Your word is a lamp to my feet and a light to my path. (Psalm 119:105)

How could I doubt the power of God's word to have this calming, settling effect on our souls, even when we do not always fully grasp every part of what it says? The book is metaphysical and mysterious. There may not be a full, rational explanation as to why it has this effect that the world can understand, but the fact remains that it brings about peace for those who earnestly practice it and pursue the One about whom it is written. The sweet irony here is that we discover He is pursuing us. According to John 6:44, "No one can come to Me unless the Father who sent Me draws him, and I will raise him up on the last day." Incredibly, though we have nothing to offer Him, He seeks to redeem us anyway. In Ephesians 2:4-6, we learn,

> But God, being rich in mercy, because of the great love with which he loved us, even when we were dead in our trespasses, made us alive together with Christ—by grace you have been saved— and raised us up with him and seated us with him in the heavenly places in Christ Jesus.

To review, I'm sitting here nodding off because I'm sleep-deprived, half-understanding the words in front of me. I can't even remember what I just read two sentences ago. But I know I feel more grounded and more secure when I have been immersed in Scripture for a time, and so I continue to do it even when I'm incredibly weak, and it turns out that the real reason I'm reading is because God has compelled me to take an interest in the things of God in the first place. This is incredible. I have done nothing to deserve this kindness. Someday, as I am drawing my last breaths, I hope someone will read Scripture to me. Surely it will settle us all.

This chapter asks how we can face hard things without living in terror, and my first and best answer is to rely upon Scripture.

This chapter asks how we can face hard things without living in terror, and my first and best answer is to rely upon Scripture. Another is to consider the fact that the anticipation of a dreaded event is almost always worse than the actual event itself. I remember one beautiful autumn day in 2009 as I was enjoying a jog through the streets of my hometown, a strange thought came to me: I was thankful that I did not know what the next day would bring. For some reason, I just had a sudden awareness that we don't want to know the future. If we knew the future, it would be impossible to enjoy the present, because there is always something looming in the future that will frighten us.

The words of Jesus in Matthew 6:34, "Therefore do not be anxious about tomorrow for tomorrow will be anxious for itself. Sufficient for the day is its own trouble." What a simple bit of profound wisdom. Only a few days after my jogging epiphany, we received that 4:00 a.m. call to come to Mom and Dad's house.

Another experience we had a decade earlier was that I had made dinner one Monday night and ended up with far more food than we needed. It was a dish I knew my mother-in-law enjoyed, and I asked Eric if he would like to take dinner out to his parents and share it with them. Never in our married life had this happened, but Betty had been recuperating at home from a diabetes-related surgery, and it seemed like a good idea to do this, so we did. We enjoyed a good visit with his parents and were so glad we had shared this meal with them. The next day Eric's oldest brother called mid-afternoon to report that their mother had passed away. She had died suddenly of congestive heart failure, completely unexpected (someone years later joked that my cooking might have been the culprit). As young thirty-somethings, these events stunned us. Neither of us had ever lost someone close. Eric and his brothers and father managed the funeral arrangements and worked together to provide a service that honored Betty as best they could while they dealt with the shock and grief, for which they could not have been prepared. Realization sank in that we cannot know what the next twenty-four hours, or even fifteen

Realization sank in that we cannot know what the next twenty-four hours, or even fifteen seconds will bring.

seconds will bring, and I'm convinced we don't want to know, either. Eric and I managed to live this long before losing one of our parents. I cannot even imagine the lives of students I've had whose parent(s) died before they even graduated. This has happened more times than I care to count, and each of these stories is heartbreaking. Some of my former senior students know the harsh reality of comfortable contentedness one minute and deep sorrow the next, having tragically lost classmates or siblings. My hospice social worker, Casie, lost her young adult brother, and wishes she had known ahead so she could say all the things that were left unsaid at the time, which is understandable. As for me, I want to leave the future just as it is: unknown.

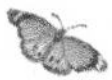

During Dad's short-lived brain cancer period, I was driving him to the cancer center for another radiation treatment. He was unsettled that day, and I absent—mindedly asked, "What's wrong?

"Brain tumor."

"Oh, I'm sorry." What was I thinking? Of course, brain tumor.

"I just wish I could get rid of this stress!" I had nothing to offer, driving in stupefied silence. "I just wish I knew what was on the other side of this thing." This time I did have an answer but knew better than to reply because no, he didn't want to know. We had been told about and had read about glioblastomas, and barring an act of God, death was certainly on the other side. I didn't know if he was referring to the radiation, the illness, Heaven, or what, but it didn't seem safe to question. He just needed to vent, and I was the unlucky recipient of his angst that day. While Dad handled his predicament honorably, he was human, and subject to the stages most people go through when grieving the inevitable loss of control. If there is a word in the English language that could capture Dad's personality, it would be that—control. This trait usually resulted in good works. He took responsibility, orchestrated events, faced challenges, and bulldozed through most obstacles with bravery. Cancer, among other life-threatening diseases, reminds us that we are not in control at all, and probably never were to begin with. Master planner and organizer though he was, if he had known what was on the other side, he couldn't have done a single thing about it.

While in hospice Dad's inner control freak surfaced again, only this time it had the three of us rolling with laughter. Disoriented, Dad asked, "What time is the funeral?" We sat in confused silence, realizing he was still trying to direct events over which he had zero control. "Oh! I gotta die first," came his serious reply to himself. Maybe it was crass to laugh so hard at this, but it was so characteristic for him to inquire about the time, and he cracked himself up as well once it occurred to him what he had said. If he is still telling stories in Heaven, I know this is one he has surely shared, getting some good laughs out of his last days on earth. Still, it remains that we don't know what's on the other side, we can't control what's there, and it might not even be any of our business!

I will trust that God is with me just as He has been all along.

If someone had told me in 2016 what would unfold in the next five years, I would have lived in fear and dread. Some of what happened truly was dreadful, but there was so much good that happened too. I endured some difficulties, but nothing was so terrible that it would have warranted crippling dread and anxiety. What lies ahead is unknown to me, and what I have read about my condition is unpleasant. However, I will trust that God is with me just as He has been all along. I will remember that this life is a vapor, and I will hold to 2 Corinthians 5:7-8, "For we walk by faith, not by sight—but we are of good courage and prefer rather to be absent from the body and to be at home with the Lord." Being the sort of people who tend toward morbid humor, it might also be true that we have some good laughs in store.

One more way to manage those moments when thinking is fragmented or emotions are chaotic is to journal. I have kept a journal for years, and if anyone were to stumble upon the decades-old stacks and begin reading, they would soon be either asleep or confused. The writing has been for myself, to help sort my thoughts and emotions about a wide variety of life issues. Consequently, they are uninteresting to anyone other than me. Dumping my scrambled thinking into the journal, I have been able to examine issues more thoughtfully, and after scratching my swirling cursive onto several pages, order and calm usually begins to emerge. Sometimes my earlier entries ended in prayer. As the years have elapsed, I notice a shift. When I was a younger woman, my journal was a collection of thoughts that moved from randomness to order as I wrote. This still holds true, but there are far less entries about whatever I'm thinking and far more prayers. I've discovered that whatever I'm thinking about usually necessitates prayer, and while the petitions might begin with self-focused requests, these give way to larger concerns that go far beyond myself. Always, as my pencil draws the entry to a close, I am relieved of my burden and refreshed once again.

In April of 2020, shortly before the surgery to remove the new masses in my abdomen, I was afraid. It was also just after Covid had shut down the world, and it seemed everything was falling apart. I was experimenting with poetic forms and wrote this sonnet in my journal, attempting to reconcile myself to mortality. The poem explains much more succinctly what I have tried to say in this chapter. It is more relevant now than before.

Final Flight

Relinquished, given over to the task
Of gliding to an earthly resting place
Descending through opaqueness, skies that mask
Terrain that we must all one day embrace.
I'm drifting, so serene, sometimes with joy—
At other times, a turbulence ensues.
My center shakes, my foe seeks to destroy
the gift (secure) of faith I cannot lose.
A fog obscures the landing, lest I see
Events I must unstintingly embrace
With gratitude, though ravaged I may be,
Because I so desire to see His face.
Equipped with nothing that would recommend
My soul, that on His mercy does depend.

Your Reflections

1. What is your biggest fear concerning your own mortality?

2. What thoughts of dread and despair spring up in your thinking, uninvited?

3. What are some healthy options that have brought you comfort in hard times before (being in nature, talking with a friend, watching a comedy, etc.)?

4. What unhealthy coping options are temptations for you (drinking, gambling, etc.)?

5. What wisdom have you gathered from others who have endured suffering—who were they and how did they handle it?

6. What has happened in your life that you're glad you didn't know about in advance?

7. What are some good things that have come or might come from your experience of suffering?

8. What Scriptures or hymns are important to you—that you cling to in difficulty?

9. How would you advise someone else to avoid negative thinking?

10. *Prayer*: Write to God about what is heavy on your heart right now, and ask Him for help and support. Give thanks for any help or support you have already received.

Chapter Four

Living While Dying

Our final work is to live meaningfully while dying.

What do we exchange in letting go of the earthly to gain the heavenly?

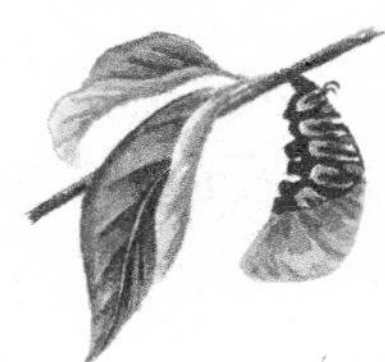

My best pal Eric (also known as my husband) and I have much in common. There is still room to say opposites attract, but for decades now we have found a workable rhythm in our marriage, managing to balance each other's strengths and weaknesses. Where he is a long-range strategic planner, I am spontaneous. Where I love working with words whether reading, writing, or speaking, he is quiet and pensive. It turns out, though, that he is more social, while I am content to live a hermit existence, busy with little projects at home in solitude. We have had lots of time to work out our complementary differences, and as old pros at marriage, we were both shocked to discover that there was anything remaining about ourselves or each other that we didn't know. We found that we both possessed a personality trait, unbeknownst to us, that would help us understand ourselves, especially as we relate to others.

A few years ago, our Sunday School class worked on a spiritual gifts study. In it were multiple surveys and graphs using many measures to identify and define them, and the class completed these eagerly, desiring to make better use of our natural God-given gifts for His kingdom. Early in the study, we found that both of us are task-oriented. Not just a little bit—we are extremely task-oriented. This was not what was so shocking to us, as we were somewhat aware of it. What was astounding was that the opposite end of the spectrum was an orientation toward people. Neither of us came close to being people-oriented. Still, we assumed this would be typical. Our instructor asked for a show of hands to reveal results, and Eric and I were the only task-oriented people in the room. Every other person in our class was people-oriented! I was stunned to find our hands the only ones in the air, and it explained so much about ourselves, our home, and why we are sometimes baffled by others' ways of doing life.

As a tasker, I have always loved to-do lists. I have notebooks full of old to-do lists that I have been hesitant to discard, because their pages of marked-off tasks represented the satisfaction with task completion. These lists detailed family birthday dinners and holidays, cleaning chores, camping trips and vacations, garden plans, and every manner of undertaking one might expect in the running of a busy household. Eric had a few of these lists as well, but his looked more like sketches and diagrams, as he often has a woodworking project or landscaping plan underway. He makes detailed drawings with notes, and these can be found tucked in every nook of the house that he has claimed as his. We had no idea that this was out of the ordinary, but we knew that most of our friends and acquaintances had television shows they watched faithfully, where our TV may go a couple of weeks without being turned on, especially in summer. We know they are busy doing worthwhile things with their lives, but we have no idea what those things are. Maybe they go to more parties? We will never know. We enjoy being busy improving our home, and we like being creative. Creatures of habit, we have always had dinner and conversation at our kitchen table together every evening, after which we do the dishes together, followed by each of us going separate directions to work on our individual projects or task lists. Then, we reconvene later in the evening and discuss whatever we completed. This might make us a couple of weirdos in the eyes of these newly discovered people-oriented creatures by which we are apparently surrounded. However, this is life the way we like it. Even through my previous bouts with cancer treatment, this routine did not waver much except on treatment weeks. Our boats were rocked, but our rudders remained undisturbed.

After the last two chemo treatments this winter, my lists vanished as I languished in my chair, too fatigued to do much more than get a shower and put on clothes. Productivity was at an all-time low. As I write, I have now rebounded some, and am back to list-making, but it is spring. Normally, those lists would be miles long and full of gardening to-dos. Now I am content to simply sit outdoors and listen to the birds. As my vigor has gradually diminished, I've had to admit that for a while, I was in the doldrums. "Doldrums" is a fantastic word. A quick glance at it usually prompts us to think of someone in a temporary funk, but it means so much more. A nautical term, it refers to weather conditions near the equator that are utterly stagnant, causing sailing ships to remain stationary. There is no breeze to billow the sail that hangs listlessly as the ship sleepily bobs in sync with the lackluster waves. The condition can last for long stretches, causing near madness in sailors whose activity level quickly mimics that of the ship. Recovering slowly and incompletely has gotten my attention. The doldrums have forced me to become reacquainted with my identity.

Those notebooks full of completed activities had served to define my roles and falsely shape my identity. I have been a busy wife, daughter, mother, grandmother, teacher, and friend. I make things and attempt to be orderly and creative. These simple descriptors were how I was accustomed to thinking about myself, and they point to *how* I have spent time. When we are busy enacting our roles, we can lose touch with Christ as our identity. It is possible to pray often and read His word but still live as if He is an accessory to our active lives. An accessory is a mere add-on, where an identity is the very heart of who we are. God will not be an accessory. When our lives become cluttered with endless tasks that usurp time and energy instead of giving each day back to Him, our priorities will get rearranged. He will determine what work we are to do, which may or may not match our self-perception. Ephesians 2:10 says, "For we are his workmanship, created in Christ Jesus for good works, which God prepared beforehand, that we should walk in them." This means we must be ready each day for anything, and anything might look like the doldrums. I have found that there is much good to be done while in the doldrums.

God will not be an accessory.

Before that discovery, though, I kept finding myself wanting to volunteer for things, wanting to be involved and active at church, and in home projects. I was dismayed at first. It was like being at a ball where everyone is in step, swirling briskly across the dance floor, but I was unable to join with either the speed or the exuberance required, then realizing I was now consigned to the perimeter, watching from afar. My friend Angela, who has late-stage cancer, is experiencing the same thing. For years, her life has revolved around her work as a middle and high school music teacher. She has built a vivacious program with robust participation and strong community support. Frequently collaborating with her husband Lex, head of the theater department in the school, their lives were unceasingly consumed with theater, music, students, and school-related activities. Weakened by cancer and treatment, and sheltering at home due to low immunity, she has found herself in the doldrums. At every opportunity, she still volunteered to work the sound booth or be involved with classes via computer screen, remaining attached to the music department for as long as possible. It was heart-wrenching for her to let go of the school, the program, and the students. She knows very well that her identity is in Christ, but she, too, has been gently escorted to the perimeter for now.

It is a new time for those of us at the perimeter of life's commotion. Most of us are familiar with chapter three of Ecclesiastes. In it, life's activities are written in poetic form using a dichotomous structure. Solomon tells us,

> There is a time for everything,
> and a season for every activity under the heavens,
> a time to be born and a time to die,
> a time to plant and a time to uproot,
> a time to kill and a time to heal,
> a time to tear down and a time to build,
> a time to weep and a time to laugh,
> a time to mourn and a time to dance,
> a time to scatter stones and a time to gather them,
> a time to embrace and a time to refrain from embracing,
> a time to search and a time to give up,
> a time to keep and a time to throw away,
> a time to tear and a time to mend,
> a time to be silent and a time to speak,
> a time to love and a time to hate,
> a time for war and a time for peace.

Solomon continues later, saying "He has made everything beautiful in its time."

For those of us in our final stretch, this is a time to slow down. A time to cocoon. A time for last things. A time to tie up loose ends. Endeavors that once consumed our attention may no longer interest us because we are undergoing a massive shift. We are decelerating, and naturally, this will have a sifting effect on the activities of ordinary life. We are still alive and have the same number of hours in the day as before, so the question often looms regarding how they should be spent. Angela and I discussed this recently, and we found commonality in our desire to spend more time in the Bible, in praying, and in strengthening family connections. Perhaps this is our new work the Father has for us, no less essential than our previous enterprises.

Gerry, an old friend and my boss from years ago who suffered from ALS, gradually lost his strength and mobility and was able to do very little in his final years, months, and weeks. He was a man of faith and an avid sports enthusiast. Formerly a college baseball athlete, he loved to play for years afterward, including co-ed leagues with friends and his wife, Aggie. For him, watching sports on television helped pass the long hours and helped him maintain contact with the activities he loved. Unlike many afflicted with ALS, he did not lose his ability to speak, and was able to enjoy the company of friends and family. Aggie recalls that he kept everyone laughing as he engaged in his usual banter, his upbeat disposition never growing bitter or self-pitying. He lived out his faith in the way he treated others, especially in his gratitude and kindness toward her, and he demonstrated the essence of Jesus in the way he showed love, grace, and passion. 1 Thessalonians 5:11 urges, "Therefore encourage one another and build each other up, just as in fact you are doing." It is no insignificant thing to acknowledge others in their good work. Gerry continued in his assignment for the Kingdom in this way until his final hour.

This beautiful verse in 2 Corinthians 2:14 assures us that no matter the season or circumstance, whether we are leading the charge or watching from the sidelines, we are still involved in Kingdom work.

> But thanks be to God, who in Christ always leads us in triumphal procession, and through us spreads the fragrance of the knowledge of him everywhere.

We have an assignment each day, regardless of the way in which it is carried out. I remind myself that while I am breathing, there are others watching my example, observing my faith, and potentially encouraged if I fulfill my purpose, which remains despite outward physical appearance. 2 Timothy 1:9 underscores the point.

> . . . who saved us and called us to a holy calling, not because of our works but because of His own purpose and grace, which He gave us in Christ Jesus before the ages began.

His purpose. His grace. At last we can rest and stop worrying that we should be doing this or that as we used to. It is neither necessary nor expected. Instead, we can lean into what's happening in our bodies and in our lives by taking a quick inventory to help clear our minds.

I remind myself that while I am breathing, there are others watching my example.

To assist toward that end, a helpful tool is found in a manual by William Bridges, *Managing Transitions*.[3] Bridges begins by explaining the difference between change and transition. "Change is situational: the move to a new site, the retirement of the founder, the reorganization of the roles on the team, the revisions to the pension plan." Transition, though, is a consequence of change. We can observe, name, and describe change. Bridges explains that all changes, even good ones such as marriages and the birth of children, new jobs, or moving to a new home have an emotional response. That emotional response is the transition. He elaborates,

> Transition . . . is psychological; it is a three-phase process that people go through as they internalize and come to terms with the details of the new situation that the change brings about.

These phases are Ending, Losing, and Letting Go.[4] Bridges seeks to help people move through what he calls the emotional wilderness of transition by identifying and detailing the three phases unique to the change. We are often unaware of these as we move through change and become stuck in emotional turmoil until we can sort it out in this way. Only then can we move on to what Bridges calls The New Beginning, and we almost never know what it's going to look like.

I had forgotten about the book until I spotted it on a bookshelf one day and it occurred to me that I should journal about the three phases to help wrap my brain around what was happening. Could I even identify what was ending, what I was losing, or what I must let go of? It was valuable to find out.

Ending

- vacations—travel is exhausting and physically difficult
- camping trips
- outings with friends and family
- yard work and planting flowers
- sewing, crafting
- hosting events and parties
- cooking our meals, grocery shopping
- personal purchases that won't benefit others in some way after I'm gone

- planning improvement projects at home
- participation in community activities
- teaching—both school and Sunday school
- being called on by others to help with projects
- being able to supervise grandchildren
- being busy and feeling productive

Most of the things are mundane elements of everyday life, all of which I have enjoyed to the fullest. They are statements of the obvious, and it is worthwhile to inventory them. They are the kinds of things that can be found on task lists. Losing, though, is different.

Losing

- the ability to do anything entertaining with/for grandchildren—role has changed from active grandparent to sick one
- the ability to work with others on projects such as helping with my daughter's wedding, Vacation Bible School at church—role as team player and helper is now gone
- leadership—decision-making role now limited to end-of-life decisions
- some friendships, quietly dissipating
- the ability to be an equal marriage partner—take more than give, which will escalate
- the ability to take care of myself later on
- eventually, everything earthly

The list above pertains mostly to roles I have played, and I am glad to see that as my fulfillment of those roles recedes, others can and will step up. Someone else will get the family together. Others will engineer family events, and they will do it with more energy and creativity than I have for a while now. My exit means that others will be empowered to enter those family-nurturing functions, and theirs are capable hands.

The only item on this list that disturbs me is being an equal marriage partner. I do not like taking more than I give, and this bothers me a lot. I don't see a way to feel better about it or to fix it, and I am nowhere near being able to accept it yet, either. For now, I must hang out with this bewilderment, with no resolution in sight. When Eric and I married, at ages twenty-two and nineteen respectively, we were straight serious about our vows. I recall wanting to keep them as traditional as possible, including lots of Scripture. We meant what we said but couldn't possibly imagine what this covenant might someday demand. Those of us who have made marriage vows and held to them with fidelity are discovering, year by year, that trouble is never far away. To be sure, there are good times, but anything can happen, any time, to steal our peace if we do not have it anchored to someone who is stronger than both of us. In other words, we are not the basis of our own marriage, because even individually we are not our own. 1 Corinthians 6:19-20 states,

> Or do you not know that your body is a temple of the Holy Spirit within you, who you have from God? You are not your own, for you were bought with a price. So glorify God in your body.

If it is true that our bodies are temples of the Holy Spirit, then together, our marriage must be based upon Him as well. Because this has been our foundation, albeit stronger at some times than others, we have been strengthened to fulfill the long-held vows.

I, ______, take you, ______, to be my (husband/wife),
to have and to hold from this day forward,
for better, for worse,

for richer, for poorer,
in sickness and in health,
to love and to cherish,
until we are parted by death.
This is my solemn vow.

These vows are, indeed, solemn. Think of the people you know whose finances are in ruins, whose kids have made terrible decisions, whose lives have been wrecked by automobile accidents, whose homes have burned to the ground, whose health has fallen apart. We foresee none of these when we stand at the altar, and even if we did, we would not understand what would be required of us. Eric and I have discovered those requirements over the years, but this end-of-life challenge is probably our hardest.

Finally, it is time to examine what I must let go.

Letting Go

- control—just an illusion anyway
- relationships—must let go of them and let them all move on with their lives without me
- roles—hard not to see myself in former roles—must let go.
- the known—everything I have ever known about reality must be relinquished
- physical body—I must separate from it

It would be hard to find anyone who didn't see the movie "Back to the Future." Protagonist Marty McFly has interfered with his destiny by meeting his future parents, and he is terrified they might not end up together due to his interference. He keeps looking at a photograph in which he fades in and out of existence, depending on how well the attraction thrives between them. While I haven't time traveled, I do have a sense of progressively vanishing. It is early yet, but I feel it, the first occurrence having been leaving the classroom.

Soon after deciding to leave the classroom, removing my personal effects from it had to be done. I wrote earlier about this, saying that after it was done, I didn't look back. While that is true, it is also true that the process of doing it made me sad. It was faster to cram those carefully selected items into boxes than it had been to thoughtfully place them around the room, but it wasn't easier. When I first took possession of this room in late 2015, it was a disaster. The previous teacher was not interested in décor, function, or organization. Furniture and posters were placed haphazardly, while files and office supplies were stuffed randomly in drawers and cabinets. She had abruptly left the classroom in November. The short-term substitute who got it functioning again told me I should have seen it then. Apparently, trash had accumulated in every nook and ungraded papers were piled high. There was little evidence that love of learning reigned in this dirty, disorganized space by either teacher or students.

Christmas Break had just begun. I had between December 17 and January 4 to get this room together, create a syllabus, and establish routines and procedures where evidently none had existed. Filled with joy at the prospect of making this a space where students would feel valued, where they could be immersed in writing projects and good literature and possibly even enjoy it, I worked feverishly, and my husband and son, Logan, pitched in for the heavy lifting. By the January deadline it wasn't beautiful, but it was organized and functional. As the months advanced, I added aesthetic touches here and there, eventually creating the learning space I envisioned from the start. The master to-do list for that endeavor had been a multi-page beast. Now, no list was necessary.

Step one: shove everything in a box and haul it home. Check.

To dismantle the room seemed irreverent; dismissing the many valued relationships, friendly conversations, and academic "aha" moments as irrelevant left me feeling vacant and stunned. Slowly wiping away the accumulated dust and pencil shavings, I thought back over the previous four-and-a-half years, reviewing all I had learned and loved and was now losing. I disassembled the coffee bar, thinking back to the students who came in for an early morning chat, or popped in between classes to pour a cup and tell me about their weekend or their break-up, show prom dress pictures or progress on their engine rebuild. The blue tissue paper flowers suspended over the reading corner came down, rustic literary décor elements were stashed, and handmade posters were rolled up.

Finally, I turned off the lights and locked the classroom door for the last time.

I thought back to the gratifying comments students made year after year, male and female, telling me they loved my classroom because it was relaxing and welcoming. Not everyone loved English, but they loved being in a space that was designed with them in mind. They had no idea what a privilege and honor it was for me to create it in the first place, or the story of how I came to get this job had been a series of small miracles. I felt somber and grieved. Eric, ever my wingman, helped me with this cheerless task. As I finished sealing boxes, he hauled them to his truck. Finally, I turned off the lights and locked the classroom door for the last time. Boxes and their contents were resettled in our home. I was not devastated, but my usually cheerful disposition was subdued for a few days, wistful that God's gift of this work was a short chapter, now ending.

This was my first concrete indicator that I would flicker out of existence sooner rather than later, but I've now had a while to get used to the idea. For those whose hard diagnoses and abrupt losses have come more suddenly, I am so sorry. Leaving what we have loved is tough to accept, and it takes time to let go. Earlier, I detailed the Ending, Losing, and Letting Go phases of navigating transition. What I didn't mention is the piece those with sudden diagnoses are missing: The Neutral Zone. Bridges explains that The Neutral Zone is the gap between Ending-Losing-Letting Go and The New Beginning.[5] The transition doesn't happen quickly or easily. Instead, he characterizes that Neutral Zone gap as being messy and sometimes disorienting.

Many people find that being in nature and/or having solitude to let the changes settle during the Neutral Zone is critical. Grieving people, whether losing a loved one or losing their own life, have a much more profound sense of loss to absorb than those targeted in Bridges's work and should not expect to simply get over it and move on, especially in cases of short notice. They may need to carve out time for their Neutral Zone experience by talking with a social worker or chaplain, taking a low-activity trip with undisturbed time to think, or asking companions to give them some quiet time to process their life-altering changes. Think beaches, nature trails, porch-sitting, or similar serene settings. I threw porch-sitting in that list because that's what it was for me. I resolved much while sitting in the sunshine on my porch rocker and it didn't cost a dime. My case has been one of slow and steady decline, with long periods of nearly normal functioning in between. I have had the luxury of absorbing my losses over time, which has helped with acceptance.

Bridges's book has helped me list and detail the simple and obvious, which isn't at all simple or obvious to people who learn they're at the end of life. It would be much more expedient to say everything is ending, we are losing everything, and we must let go of everything. But the lived experience isn't as simple as that. To imagine each aspect of our lives as transient is an exercise in acceptance.

In the Old Testament, we have an example in Job, who could have compiled quite an impressive list of his own losses too. Our circumstances may not be as catastrophic as his were, but the losses are just as personal. It is important to note that God restored everything to Job many times over, and He does this for us, too, in eternity. Our losses are nothing in comparison to what we gain in the life that is to come. In John 14:1-3, Jesus promises,

> Let not your hearts be troubled. Believe in God; believe also in me. In my Father's house are many rooms. If it were not so, would I have told you that I go to prepare a place for you? And if I go and prepare a place for you, I will come again and will take you to myself, that where I am you may be also.

This, we can never lose. Paul puts it concisely, "For me, to live is Christ, to die is gain," in Philippians 1:21. It is for us, too. All His people have everything to gain in a short while.

In his book *Heaven*, Randy Alcorn does a meticulous job citing every Scripture reference to Heaven, describing what the Bible tells us in-depth about our true home.[6] The 533-page book is filled with scriptural answers to questions I obviously cannot describe here, but any Christian with a Bible will find plenty of confirmation that there is a Heaven that awaits, and plenty of evidence that it will be mind-blowingly fantastic. Our losses will be instantly obliterated by the glory that is to come.

God restored everything to Job many times over, and He does this for us, too, in eternity.

Tom, Casie, and Beth, my wonderful hospice team, have shared what sometimes happens when believers are dying. Most die with peaceful expressions, but some burst into huge smiles, reaching up toward something in their final seconds. They are taking their first steps into their New Beginning, something we cannot fathom until it is our time. This is a small glimpse of the glorious hope that awaits!

Your Reflections

1. Do you consider yourself task-oriented or people-oriented, and how can you tell?

2. How have you been spending your time and energy since your terminal diagnosis?

3. In your situation, what is ending?

4. What are you losing?

5. What must you let go of?

6. How has your identity been falsely shaped by your roles and activities?

7. If you could choose a perfect Neutral Zone for yourself, what would it be? If it isn't feasible, what kind of Neutral Zone might be achievable for you?

8. What do you most look forward to in Heaven?

9. As you look back to the date of your diagnosis, in what ways can you sense God's hand in your story?

10. *Prayer:* Write to God about whatever thoughts this chapter has prompted in you. Thank Him for all the ways in which you have been supported.

Chapter Five

Chinks in the Armor

Deception is always ready to devour what faith has built up.

How do we live in the world without being of the world?

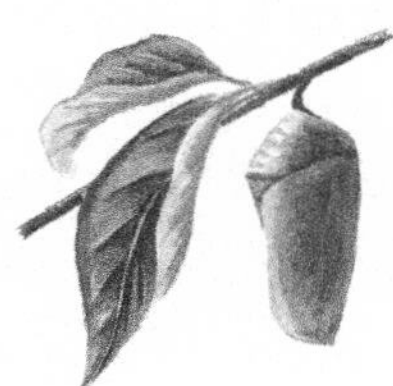

To live in the world without being of it: what does that mean? Are there people among us, hidden masters who have transcended the world and live on a higher plane of existence, tucked away in monastic seclusion? Looking at what the Bible says about this needs to come before anything else in this chapter.

- Praying for His disciples, Jesus says to His Father, "They are not of the world, just as I am not of the world" (John 17:16).
- The Apostle Paul exhorts the Romans, "Do not be conformed to this world, but be transformed by the renewal of your mind, that by testing you may discern what is the will of God, what is good and acceptable and perfect" (Romans 12:2).
- John's epistle reminds, "We know that we are from God, and the whole world lies in the power of the evil one" (1 John 5:19).

These and many other verses indicate that the world is a fallen place whose inhabitants are ruled by sin. God's people are to be separate, but this doesn't mean we can no longer enjoy anything in the world. God created it, after all, and there is much to be enjoyed. To put it simply, we are to cease striving in the way the rest strive and to build our lives on conforming to God's will, desiring to please Him. It should be noted, too, that we cannot accomplish this on our own any more than we achieved salvation on our own. To build my life on conformity to His will, reading His word faithfully has been essential for me. Without knowledge of the Word, we are on our own, doing what is right in our own eyes, which leads us straight to self-satisfaction, exactly where we don't want to be.

During the time of the Judges, when there was no king in Israel or Judah, the people did their best to rule as they saw fit. One bad decision led to another, with atrocities mounting and righteousness spiraling ever downward. Judges 21:25 concludes with the sad statement, "In those days there was no king in Israel. Everyone did what was right in his own eyes." People ruled without seeking God. The account of what happened is sobering, as it always is when we do what is right in our own eyes, yet that has never stopped us whether we are kings or commoners.

We desire to shed every vestige of our earthly striving in preparation for our homecoming.

In a book about facing death, a chapter on living in the world without being of the world is deserved. As we review our lives, we may see how fully immersed in the world we were, and now more than ever, we desire to shed every vestige of our earthly striving in preparation for our homecoming. For a blessed few, their entire lives have been lived with this eternal perspective. The rest of us have come to it later, taking much more time to understand the need for consistent Scripture reading and prayer, seeking the community of believers, and desiring to live in the shadow of His wings. And lest we think that because we are near the end, we can relax our spiritual vigilance, neglecting Scripture or forgetting prayer, we are mistaken. The one who prowls about like a roaring lion seeking whom he might devour does not care how many days we have left on earth. Now is the time to put on the full armor of God like never before. Prey that is already down is easiest to overcome, and a terminal diagnosis tends to take us down pretty quickly.

Easy prey aren't in short supply. Those downed by illness or other calamity make for good feasting, but those who are fueled by the world's praise for achievement are poised for an easy take-down as well. This forthcoming account details just how easy it is to fall away, something that happens to many of us. I share it to be transparent about my own falling away, in hopes that others may catch a glimpse of themselves and their own parallel stories. It is always amazing to me how patient and gracious God was in allowing me to run the wrong direction, straight into a dark forest, only showing me the way back when I was finally ready to admit I was lost. I am thankful He did this well before the end of my life. Perhaps you have had an experience like mine.

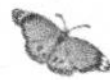

In 2005, I was offered a job in the large school district where I already worked. The offer was quite unexpected, and I did not feel prepared to take it but did so anyway against my better judgment. My fragile ego was flattered, and the pay increase was tempting, so I took the dive. It was a promotion involving administrative work and large projects requiring immaculate organizational skills. The work involved coordinating in-service time for teachers, facilitating learning labs for large groups of varied staff on a regular basis, coordinating staff development, providing training modules for college-to-classroom teachers as well as training the mentors who would shepherd them. It also included supervising the work of teachers who provided support at the campus level, and my main role was to mentor and support them as they, in turn, did this for teachers in their buildings. Last, our office was responsible for coordinating and tracking teacher licensure data for the whole district.

I was determined to make a success of it, but it proved to be so much more work than I ever imagined. There was no way I could complete everything to a high standard because the workload was huge, and much of the skill set required was new to me. I loved working directly with the teachers themselves and enjoyed bringing everyone together for the learning labs. I also believed strongly in the importance of mentoring brand-new teachers. The problem with the mismatch between myself and the work was that it required so much communication across so many levels, mostly via email. So much orchestration was required to keep all these plates spinning. It was mind-boggling. I had envisioned spending lots of time being among people, facilitating learning sessions and mentoring. What it ended up being was an endless grind in front of the computer. The second year began with a pay raise and a more ostentatious title, which did put a shine on the situation for a few minutes, but it dulled quickly. I say all this to illustrate the point that when there was an opportunity for something interesting in my day, I sopped it up it like a giant sponge.

That interesting part of the workday was the amount of reading required to stay abreast of research and trends. To that end, I participated in many book studies with colleagues. These learning-focused sessions led to good friendships, which made the studies even more engaging. Often, 6:00 a.m. cafe meetings were our way of squeezing them into the workday. It was bright and early, but we didn't mind, being joyfully wrapped up in pastries, coffee, and conversation. Readings were always focused on topics related to improving classroom practice, our passion. Part of this study branched into ways to increase teachers' consciousness, or self-awareness in the classroom. This characteristic in teachers, when increased, leads to better classroom success for teachers and students.

Teachers who have the ability to take an aerial view of the classroom, not just observing the students, but observing themselves with full awareness of the impact they are having on the classroom climate, are very effective because they can modify their own behavior to get better results from students. This trait is called "consciousness," and surprisingly, not all teachers have it. Not all people have it. Simply put, it is the ability to see oneself and understand one's own impact on others in any given situation. Some researchers call this "withitness," but consciousness was the term we were accustomed to using. These details are important to explain because it was at this juncture that I wandered into strange territory.

"Consciousness" is the ability to see oneself and understand one's own impact on others in any given situation.

I found this concept of consciousness so intriguing and began to delve into it on my own, seeking to understand the mystery of consciousness to understand why some are oblivious to it while others are masterful at it. I wondered, could this be taught? Can people be coached to increase it? Is it innate or learned?

While the readings within our professional book studies pertained to helping schools improve, my own personal studies of consciousness diverged drastically. Pretty soon I was reading psychology books explaining consciousness, and the notion that there are differing levels of it among humans. According to this theory, anyone could be mapped on a logarithmic scale of human consciousness, and the possibility exists that they could be helped to move up the scale with appropriate support.

I found the idea of helping people develop stronger consciousness so intriguing, because I had seen it result in much better classroom practice. I believed and still believe there is something important about this. God created this intangible thing called a consciousness, and growing it is quite helpful to people to become more self-aware, which leads to better rapport with others. However, right next to the beautiful flower of truth grows the invasive weed that looks deceptively like it, winding around it and mimicking its leaf patterns, escaping the gardener's notice until it has become so entangled among the flowers that removing is difficult to do without killing the flower as well. The truth about helping people develop self-awareness soon became suffocated by the weeds of Consciousness Evolution.

The idea of Consciousness Evolution is that humanity can increase its vibration, and all of society can gradually improve, or evolve over time. This is not the same concept I had initially studied, but it was a step further, and I went there. I was so deeply underwater in this study that I didn't come up for air long enough to stop and think, to see that humanity wasn't improving all on its own at all. I did not notice that this theory of Consciousness Evolution discarded the notion of sin, which was seen as irrelevant because society's problems could instead be explained in terms of low consciousness. If our only real problem is low consciousness, we only need to raise our consciousness and help others to do so too, evolving our consciousness together. No sin. No repen-

Next to the beautiful flower of truth grows the invasive weed that looks deceptively like it.

tance necessary. Nothing to confess.

Somehow, I missed the giant red flag. If sin doesn't exist, there is no need for a redeemer. Bluntly, if our consciousness is evolving on its own, we don't need Jesus. He need not have bothered with all that business on the cross since we are so sure we've got this. If we don't need Jesus, then nothing in the Bible is relevant either, aside from a bit of wisdom and history it offers.

How easily my reading had crept, little by little, into a dark forest of deception. I remember thinking that surely Consciousness Evolution has to be the same thing as sanctification, where God sanctifies us over time. I reasoned that Psychology explains it one way, and the Bible explains it another way. I remember relating this "revelation" to others, who seemed to agree. I hope I didn't share these faux pearls of wisdom with very many people. They were heretical, and spreading heresy is not very popular with God.

My biggest failure was that I failed to realize that sanctification is based upon our prior justification by faith in Jesus Christ, who made the ultimate sacrifice for our sin. There is no sanctification without Christ. Nowhere in Scripture does God cause people's consciousness to evolve, and nowhere does it evolve on its own. That escaped my attention as well. Even looking outside Scripture, there is no worldly evidence that we are evolving, either. A quick survey of society confirms that.

Trying to merge this new learning with what I knew about the Bible, I was perilously unaware of the term or concept of syncretism. The Oxford English Dictionary defines syncretism as the amalgamation of different religions, cultures, or schools of thought. Its example sentence reads, "Interfaith dialogue can easily slip into syncretism." An example of syncretism would be Chrislam, which seeks to unify Christianity and Islam. It sounds inclusive and positive to blend them. To find synthesis .

. . to bring together. Syncretism can sound good and feel good, but that doesn't mean it is good. Both of these faiths contain tenets that cannot be reconciled. It isn't negative to say so. It is simply the truth that they do not merge.

There are many other examples of syncretism, and what I was doing on my own was syncretistic; I was trying to blend Christianity with this idea of Consciousness Evolution, not really a religion, but a theory within spiritual psychology. Synthesizing that which cannot be synthesized is quickly explained by saying that puzzle pieces from two different puzzles cannot fit together to make a coherent picture. That didn't stop me.

Syncretism: The amalgamation of different religions, cultures, or schools of thought. (Oxford English Dictionary)

I wrongly saw the blending of Christianity and Consciousness Evolution as an affirmation of truth in both systems of thought rather than seeing what it actually was: diametrically opposed viewpoints that cannot be blended without compromising truth.

Compromising truth is nothing new. My thoughts were neither original nor profound. They were simply confused, and this kind of confusion has a long history. It is called Gnosticism, a centuries-old way of thinking that promotes the idea that there is hidden knowledge to be discovered which compels the seeker to unearth ever-emerging mysteries. This was the tone present in the reading into which I continued to sink. Like a glimmering mirage on a hot desert highway, Gnostic deception beckons by degree. Read this book to discover X, enroll in this mystery school to learn about Y. I had never heard of a mystery school, but the monthly magazines I was reading were full of ads for them. Week-long retreats in beautiful locations, for a sizeable fee, would yield an enlightened consciousness for the registrants and in turn, increase the consciousness vibration of the whole world. I thought the ads were hokey; there was a snake-oil quality about them, and for that reason, the question lingered as to whether the entire sum of this ideology might also be suspect. Could it be? There are educational institutions built upon these notions, so could they really be so wrong? Still, these slick but silly ads tugged at my conscience. They were full of imagery portraying crystals, the Egyptian eye, pyramids, and other such New Age trappings. Hours upon hours of my reading on consciousness was suddenly thrown under the light of suspicion by a few overplayed advertisements. Was the whole business just a bunch of New Age nonsense? It was beginning to look that way. I was never fully convinced of its truth, though I did have four toes in the water with a fifth one hovering.

Looking back, I recognize myself in 2 Timothy 3:6-7, which discusses godlessness in the last days. "... among them are those who creep into households and capture weak women, burdened with sins and led astray by various passions, always learning and never able to arrive at a knowledge of the truth." No unsavory character had crept into our household, but my stacks of books had strongly influenced me and had overtaken most of my thinking. I was spending so much time mired in reading, working, and studying that it seemed the harder I worked, the less I accomplished.

The hidden truth (somewhat hidden even from me) was that my identity was falsely defined by achievement and credentials. I was obsessed with learning so that I could prove to myself that I was not dumb. Years of probable attention-deficit issues had convinced me that I was, so it was a continual battle to prove to myself otherwise. Many people describe their falling away with stories of alcoholism, substance abuse, extramarital affairs, and outwardly obvious addictions. I had none of these. But anything can become an unhealthy fixation if done to an extreme degree and for the wrong reasons.

These academic pursuits may have appeared scholarly on the outside, but they were more accurately rooted in a self-centered quest for perfection. I sought to create this scholarly identity rather than recognizing the one I already had: the image of God.

Eric and I still retained our Christian faith, but our commitment was weak, and we quit attending church. Eric felt more connected to God when working outdoors, and our teenaged kids were fine with skipping church.

Compounding my confusion was the academic work I was doing as I completed a master's degree in School Leadership, aiming to enter a doctoral program after that. In these readings and discussions, I absorbed postmodern ideas, embracing the notion that learning is a social construct, and that truth and meaning are defined together in community.

Anything can become an unhealthy fixation if done to an extreme degree and for the wrong reasons.

I was unaware that the deeper, logical progression of this thinking would ultimately claim that truth is a subjective construct that differs in individuals. In other words, truth is not self-existent; people create truth. This was the implication, and at first, it sounded reasonable to me. Your truth, my truth. Each of us has a different truth based upon lived experiences. This sounds reasonable to so many people because it feels inclusive. It allows us to say, "You do you, and I'll do me." This is an avenue for us to coexist, to go along so we can get along. Getting along is a high ideal in a culture that does not understand how to engage in civil discourse. We have forgotten how to discuss ideas without disagreement becoming a personal assault. Nowadays, we are triggered by disagreement, so we must avoid it. We dislike discord so much that we will sacrifice truth to achieve a false peace.

Peace is false if we must hide our objections for fear of being canceled. I object to the notion that we can each have our own truth. Are serial killers Ted Bundy and Jeffrey Dahmer allowed to live according to their own truths? If so, how could they be held responsible for "crimes"? "Crimes" would be "criminal" according to someone else's truth. So, whose truth rules?

No, it was not a workable theory, and I didn't care how many credentialed geniuses said so. Reason forced me to reject postmodernism. Finally, the scales fell from my eyes when I heard a speaker discussing postmodern thought, and he asked, "If you say there is no such thing as absolute truth, how can I believe that to be absolutely true?" The whole notion was a lie, and I was saturated with its doctrines. My speech and writing dripped its counterfeit verbiage as I sought to graft still more incompatible ideas into my Christian foundation, essentially cultivating a "Christianity" of my own making.

I was never that rebellious person who refused to believe the gospel. I was the opposite, believing everything and struggling to synthesize it all into one cohesive whole; an overarching truth that encompassed the gospel, postmodernism, and Gnosticism. How had I slithered into this tawdry throne, making myself the exalted judge of truth and falsehood? I didn't feel self-important. Nevertheless, I was my own god, worshiping a golden calf of my own making. I knew the gospel but was theologically ignorant and spiritually blind. Paul cautions the early Christians in Corinth two thousand years ago of the very same error, saying "But I am afraid that as the serpent deceived Eve by his cunning, your thoughts will be led astray from a sincere and pure devotion to Christ" (2 Corinthians 11:3). How quickly a bit of unsound reading and undiscerning study can alter one's course.

My thinking was by now a cauldron of dissonance. These corrosive ideas, together with overwork, began to chafe at my conscience. With total clarity, I remember exhaustedly driving to the last of the 6:00 a.m. book talks. Five minutes from my destination, words came flying at me from nowhere I could identify. Unmistakably, the words, "What you are doing is wrong!" slammed into my brain. In an instant, I knew what was wrong: the long work hours were deteriorating my commitment to home and family. The reading I was doing opposed the gospel. The friendships surrounding work were expiring. I loved every one of these people I was surrounded with, from the university to the workplace, and I still respect them. But our commonality had run its course. "What you are doing is wrong!" applied to my allegiance to these dear people too.

Unmistakably, the words, "What you are doing is wrong!" slammed into my brain.

I believed then as well as now that the thunderbolt message I had while driving was from God. I could not respond with anything but deference to Him. I had kowtowed to everyone in the perceived power structure at work, but had not been obedient to God Himself. Until now. I replied that my life would be His to do with as He determined best, beginning right now. This turned out to be one of the most pivotal moments of my entire life. It began with a word that I would have found repulsive at that time: obedience. Nearing the stoplight where my friends waited just beyond at Panera, I wondered how the morning book talk would unfold.

Soon seated with my chocolate croissant, coffee, and books, I was surprised to feel a complete absence of delight in that day's discussion.

My friends were full of their usual fun but seemed not to notice my distance. We were somehow separated by an invisible bubble that had not existed before, and now peering in from the outside, I was simultaneously saddened but filled with peace and contentment. Outwardly, I nodded with feigned interest while inwardly, I marveled at my miraculous and sudden disinterest in anything at all being discussed.

1 Corinthians 4:33 reminds us " . . . God is not a God of confusion but of peace," and it became real to me later at the office that morning. Entering my beautiful office for another day of computer screen gazing, I felt zero energy for the work. I stood at the window, gazing west and pondering what to do. The clouds were dissipating; gray, miasmic streaks dissolving, floating apart placidly. I was struck that the hazy, overcast sky was parting to reveal clear blue depths just as my confusion was melting away to reveal discernible truth. I knew I was done. I didn't know what was next. I didn't care.

My thorough absorption in work and study would need to dissipate just as the clouds were doing outside my window. I needed to re-examine priorities and re-establish boundaries. It was time to re-center everything on God, home, and family.

My plan was to complete the contract, which meant I had seven more months of drudgery to go. Thankfully, that seven months is far behind me now. Toward the end of it, I started to feel anxious about my next step even though I had handed it to God. Trust and faith faltered, and every Christian reader knows why. I was not surrounded by a faith community and not reading the Bible. My prayers contained some thanksgiving but were mostly full of pleading. Nowhere was there praise. Despite my obvious weakness, I did begin to perceive a renewal as I depended more and more on God. How merciful He is, that he would take my paltry prayer life as it was and still breathe new life into me, a lost sheep sure of its own footing even as it stumbled into every ravine.

I had a "Shazam!" moment here. It turns out that depending on my own strength was the very thing causing the exhaustion to begin with. Depending on my own wisdom led me to make wrong choices. What on earth had happened? I used to pray all the way to work and listen to praise songs often when I first began this work with its thirty-minute commute. Those days were long gone, and prayer time had turned into listening to audiobooks. Not a moment could be wasted without the fixation on learning.

I would like to say that I realized I was lost, found my way back out of the forest, and recommitted to Christianity anew. That isn't at all what happened. I did nothing and God did it all. His words drew me back, and they were not to be resisted. He had allowed me to wander in all this fervent, pointless study until I had myself so entangled that I no longer recognized my life, then He gently led me back to it, where I discovered there was much rebuilding to do.

Every Bible-reading Christian knows Proverbs 3:5-6,

> Trust in the LORD with all your heart, and do not lean on your own understanding. In all your ways acknowledge him, and he will make straight your paths.

This verse could be the title of every chapter in this book. If I had a tattoo, this would be it. My own "wisdom" has led me to some ridiculous places. How liberating it was to relinquish control to God. While it sounds as if this happened all at once, it didn't. Fully relinquishing control, then depending on God, took a few years as He revealed in small bits where I needed to let go. Even after the first steps, though, I knew this new direction was right. That's where I was in these last weeks of work. They flew by as I prepared to leave. Then, I had the following dream:

Walking down a hazy corridor, I was escorted from behind by two beings that I could not see. They led me to a room full of people I did not know then closed the door and left, but this was not intimidating; I like meeting new people. I attempted to initiate conversation with several of them, but no one would respond to my friendly efforts. I moved closer to my new companions to get a better look at them and saw with horror that they were bent over at odd angles with their backs split down the middle like cicada shells. These were not people. They were husks of people who had left their bodies! It did not seem that the people were dead. They simply were empty husks.

Looking for a quick exit, I turned for the door but found that it had dissolved into a solid wall. There was no exit. Glancing frantically around the room, I saw a window and raced over to it. The solid glass pane was several inches thick, and through it, I could see that the room I was in was adjacent to several empty rooms with windows just like this one that all lined up visually, like windows separating train cars. These adjacent rooms were empty, but I could see movement in the furthest one, and peering closer, I could tell these were my co-workers and friends. I pounded the window with clenched fists to no avail; no one could hear me through the succession of thick glass panes. Then I awoke.

These were not people. They were husks of people who had left their bodies!

What a disturbing dream! What did it mean? I was separated from my friends and stuck in a room full of husk-people. The dream nagged at me for days, but its meaning, and I was sure there was one, eluded me. The contract ended, I packed my office, and the work was complete. I began working hard at launching my next venture, and often felt lonely and lost, as I had no one with whom to share ideas, brainstorm, or collaborate. One night not long after this transition I was asleep and began dreaming of two beings escorting me to . . . .OH NO. Not this dream again!

. . . the same room. Same husk-people. Same disappearing door. Same thick window. But now, the dream picked up where it left off. Defeated after pounding uselessly on the window, I plopped down on a bench next to one of the husks. For the first time, I noticed somber music that made me feel relaxed and sleepy. My eyes slid shut as my body drifted into a hunched-over position, and I realized as I wilted that I was about to become a husk, too. This filled me with dread, but I was powerless to fight it.

Immediately I discovered that I had floated free of my body and was able to see from a new vantage point as I ascended and then, looking up, I saw that there was no ceiling! There had never been a ceiling; the top of the room was open the entire time, and I had not known it. Flying straight up and out of the dreary room, I fluttered over the tops of adjacent rooms. I could see my colleagues and friends busy at work, chatting and laughing. They were oblivious to my presence as I flew far overhead, but I waved goodbye to them anyway. The act of waving caught my attention because what waved was not a hand or arm. It was a small, gray, dove-like wing. I was a little bird, flying away from these grim, smothering rooms, and now I swooshed through the air, light and free. The second dream made much more sense.

God guides with certainty the moment we let go of the reins.

The dream was comforting to me because it revealed that wherever I was going was a good place, and my time in the previous one had now expired. I could see that I wouldn't miss it, and I had the sense that even though I was flying freely, there was a more important, much bigger Being guiding my flight. Maybe it's foolish to be comforted by a dream. It happened fifteen years ago, but I remember every detail like it was last night. Most of my dreams are nonsensical and quickly forgotten, but rarely, one like this speaks to specific concerns in my life. Because I have the Scriptures at hand for all the inspiration needed, dreams are not a central feature of my Christian walk. I do not seek them out or delve into dream interpretation at all. Being a simple-minded creature, I'm probably not going to get it if the message isn't blatantly obvious. This dream has come to mind again because it seems to have application still, as another transition is before me. This work-related episode and its subsequent dream yielded much instruction for me that still applies.

I was only forty-three at that time and had not yet recognized the pattern that every time we experience closure, God is teaching us something. I learned that change is continuous and unpredictable. I learned how to let doors close on their own and prayerfully wait for the next one to open without pushing too hard or trusting in my own strength. I learned that seeking God before taking new steps is the best course; He guides with certainty the moment we let go of the reins. When I trust Him, sometimes my intuition increases, and I have a much better sense of how to move into the unknown. That's not the norm, though. What usually happens is that I have no idea what's happening at all, but more seasoned Christians have taught me to trust even more, knowing He is doing all the work. Experience bears out that they are right. There is a nineteenth-century hymn[7] that comes to mind; sometimes those seasoned Christians who advise do so from centuries past:

When we walk with the Lord in the light of His Word,
  What a glory He sheds on our way!
While we do His good will, He abides with us still,
  And with all who will trust and obey.

Obey? The very word spears hotly through rigid, prideful necks unyoked to authority. I can make the accusation because I've been a leading expert on the topic, and I know just how the notion of obedience grates against pride. How countercultural this is, too. Yet every time I have trusted God in obedience rather than trusting myself or others, He makes things happen in ways I could never have predicted. We experience the truth of Psalm 37:5, "Commit your way to the Lord; trust in him, and he will act," yet what does the world advise? Listen to your heart. Be true to yourself. Feel good about who you are. Live your best life. And my personal (un)favorite: You are enough. Living in the world tells us that we are at the center of our own worlds, possessing wisdom in our inmost parts if we could only slow down long enough to find it. We do intensive self-care, engage in self-reflection, seek self-fulfillment, build self-esteem, desire self-actualization, carve out me-time.

Someone I know wisely said, "You know, you can go to seed on that stuff." I had gone to seed. A plant that goes to seed gets long and spindly, its weak stalk expending energy to support seeds rather than strengthening or beautifying the existing plant. I'm not suggesting we should abandon taking care of ourselves. It is necessary to engage in a certain amount of self-care. Like everything else, though, the focus on self can easily become out of balance and become little more than self-indulgent navel gazing. Looking up, there is a much richer existence to be found!

Having left the job, time to read my Bible was reclaimed, and Scriptures leapt off the pages with dazzling beauty:

> For we are His workmanship, created in Christ Jesus for good works, which God prepared beforehand that we should walk in them. (Ephesians 2:10)

Our lives have meaning and purpose that He has prepared for us!

> Therefore, whether you eat or drink, or whatever you do, do all to the glory of God. (1 Corinthians 10:31)

Every part of our lives, even the small details, are significant and God sees them!

> But we all, with unveiled face, beholding as in a mirror the glory of the Lord, are being transformed into the same image from glory to glory, just as by the Spirit of the Lord. (2 Corinthians 3:18)

This is our true identity!

Truth resounded on every page of the Bible. When I had been living in the world unaware and being wholeheartedly part of it, I would have dismissed this Biblical wisdom, aligning more closely with the maxim, "God helps those who help themselves."

Benjamin Franklin is often credited with the saying, but its origin goes " . . . all the way back to ancient Greece . . . the actual English version of this quote we use today was first penned by Algernon Sydney, an English politician who lived in the 1600s," writes Clarence L. Hayes, Jr. for Christianity.com.[8] Unsurprisingly, Sydney would have been marinating in the world of rebirthed Greek ideals, steeped in humanistic thought such as Protagoras's worldly wisdom that "Man is the measure of all things." Such counterfeit wisdom has been magnified and glorified in the information age, distilled into easily digestible memes. Were it not for those words spearing my conscience on that early morning drive, I would have continued to value the worldly wisdom over antiquated Biblical notions of reality. Yet those antiquated notions, when examined, reveal timeless truth to which the adherents of humanism are both ignorant and hos-

Every part of our lives, even the small details, are significant and God sees them!

tile. It is possible for a paradigm to change in an instant, as happened to me.

During a growth spurt in my otherwise slow spiritual development, I set out to make a vision board. This was when everyone I knew was attempting to manifest their visions by representing them pictorially, inspired by the hot new book at the time. Like a silly frog befriending another new snake, I read the book and watched its complementary video, still not always shrewd enough to beware Gnosticism's kaleidoscopic, repackaged allure. But still, I didn't want to embrace the notion that I could manifest my destiny, knowing that to be in direct opposition to God's word. Instead, I wanted to create a vision board, but consult God about what He would have me do.

The board's design emerged in my imagination as I assembled my craft supplies: I wanted it to be circular, with wedges radiating out from the center representing different facets of my life. At the center, I would place God. Now this was a problem. Pictures of God are nonexistent, so I made an Alpha symbol, colored it, cut it out, and placed it at the center of the large cardboard circle. Ideas began to flow as to what would emanate from the center, but they were interrupted by another vision in my imagination: an Omega symbol. I designed it like the Alpha one and fastened it to the board, then in a flash of insight, saw that there was nothing more to do. The board was done.

I set out to make a vision board.

If God is the beginning and end, and if my life is submitted to Him, I have no idea what will emanate from the center because I'm not controlling it. To declare this visioning project finished was radical, completely defying the advice in my large collection of self-help books, and entirely at odds with the book I had been reading. These books were soon relegated to the dumpster, as was my vision board. I laughed as I chucked them into it and slammed the blue plastic lid, amused by the sudden U-turn that had just transpired in my brain. Apparently, my mom had been praying again.

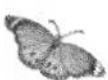

There is nothing wrong with making plans or envisioning a future. Both of my parents did, and if they hadn't, our lives would have turned out much differently. They both discovered in their youth that if anything good is to happen, they must initiate it. If family patterns of alcoholism and impulsive decision-making were to end, they would have to break the cycle, and they did. They were young in their faith, and their decision-making had more to do with survival, and with creating a life together that would not look like the lives they had left behind in their childhood homes. They married at sixteen and seventeen. As they matured in their faith, especially my mother, they desired that our family be rooted in the Christian faith, and from that time on, God shaped the direction our family took, in small increments. She was no longer of the world, and that changed everything. I thought of her influence as I worked on my vision board.

When I glued the alpha and the omega in the center of the circle, then stopped the project, my whole perspective had shifted. I did not ask God to help me with my plans. I asked God to use me as desired to enact HIS plans. When our lives are fully yielded to God, the difference between living in the world and being of the world become that plain to us. When we realize God is trustworthy, even when we don't understand what He is doing, He shields us with His peaceful presence. A hard test of this trust came when one of our grandchildren needed surgery on his skull at one year old, then again at five years old. It was hard not to worry, though eventually he healed and is now strong and healthy. In every crisis, God is my anchor, and He stabilized me with peace even when I received my own worst diagnosis.

Because we seek to please Him first, we make different choices about everything we think, say, and do. This orientation causes us to choose with discernment what our eyes and ears will be exposed to. I would even say our definition of "fun" changes! In addition, we find ourselves wanting to talk about the Lord and what He has done for us. We can do this when among other Christians, and it is so refreshing to be able to share our zeal for Christ. Some, though, regard us as extremists, neither understanding the source of our joy nor able to share in it. The gospel is an annoyance to some, and what a tragedy; they will never experience the peace and freedom we have in Christ. They are of the world, relying upon the culture for meaning and purpose. Perhaps they will make a U-turn, too. That is my prayer. Proverbs 14:12 states, "There is a way that seems right to a man, but its end is the way to death." I have shared with friends that God allowed me to dangle over the abyss for a while before snatching me safely away. I don't know why He did, but I am thankful.

In His high priestly prayer, found in John 17, Jesus prays for His disciples before He is arrested. He pleads with the Father on their behalf, saying, " . . . the world has hated them because they are not of the world, just as I am not of the world. Sanctify them in the truth; your word is truth." For those who belong to the world, the gospel sounds ridiculous. According to 1 Corinthians 1:18, "For the word of the cross is folly to those who are perishing, but to us who are being saved it is the power of God." It took a while, but I am now glad to be thought a fool, engaging in folly, completely ridiculous for the sake of the gospel.

Since 2012, Eric and I have regularly attended church again. By the time of my cancer diagnosis in 2017, we were not strangers to the notion of being in the world but not of it. However, cancer has brought me to the edge of the cliff. The prospect of impending death will do that. I care less and less each day about being of the world. Many in my colon cancer Facebook group express the very same thinking. We are intrigued and delighted by what awaits, feeling the transience of the world ever more acutely.

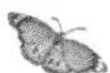

What does it mean to not be "of the world?" John the Baptist certainly wasn't. The Old Testament Prophets weren't either. Jesus absolutely wasn't. He still grew up learning carpentry skills, and apparently enjoyed feasting at weddings and hanging out with His friends. He just did everything for God's glory rather than self-gratification. His activities might have looked similar to others', but He did them with a different purpose in mind. Jesus likely did not make a vision board because He would already have known the Alpha and Omega is always at the center of everything.Those of us who follow Him desire to do the same, to put Him at the center. Our work looks ordinary but is done with a different purpose in mind.

Jesus likely did not make a vision board because He would already have known the Alpha and Omega is always at the center of everything.

Beginning with the failed cut-and-paste project that wound up in the dumpster, my life changed gradually. In small increments, fragments of dross fell away in the form of unproductive habits and thought patterns, and ways of handling conflict. The fragments continue to fall; He is not finished with me.

When self is at the center, we are blind to it. Our understanding is darkened. When God changes us, we recoil at the realization, horror-struck at the depth of our self-centeredness. We cannot make this realization on our own. Others cannot get us to see it, either. God Himself causes us to change from being temporally oriented to eternally minded. 1 Corinthians 3:7 explains, "So then neither the one who plants nor the one who waters is anything, but God who causes the growth." We can thank Him for gently showing us who we really are, then again for changing us, rearranging us from the inside out. Over time, my desire to please God grew stronger than the desire to be liked and respected by other humans, and He changed my heart of stone so that I might like and respect them with no self-interest, and without worrying about what they think of me. Another miracle.

When I say cancer brought me to the edge of the cliff, I mean this quest to please God has become more complete. This seems to have happened on its own. I know I didn't initiate it. The best explanation is found in Philippians 2:13: "For it is God who is at work in you, both to will and to work for His good pleasure." I don't know if this is true for all Christians who find themselves near the end of their lives, but for me, much that could be categorized as entertainment now is dreadfully boring. It is certain I did not make that mind shift happen. He has changed my interests, desires, and attitudes. I wish it hadn't taken cancer to make this happen. It is a secret joy, though, to be in the world yet not of it. It is like when we are sitting serenely at a cozy fire on a cold, wintry night with the wind raging outside, but instead of warming ourselves fireside, we carry the fire within us, and are continually warmed by its glow.

This was unknown to me before when I was busy jogging on the treadmill of achievement and acquisition. If I could go back to my thirty-or-forty-something self, I would say to stick with being a schoolteacher, stay in church, take care of family and home, and forget earning extra degrees and certificates and seeking to be a professional whatever. Enjoy reading your books but be more selective and spend time every day in your Bible. Seek God wholeheartedly and choose your friends accordingly. Someday when your life ends, you will want to have spent your time on what mattered. This is not to say that hard work and achievement don't matter. I am so proud of friends and family who strive and work hard to achieve their goals. But I also know that this can become an all-consuming effort, and it doesn't deserve as much of our time and attention as I gave it. Lose what's unimportant. Let go of the pointless activities and attachments. In the end, all that matters is how you honored God and how you treated your family first and others second. Paraphrasing James Dobson of Focus on the Family, my hospice chaplain Tom recently remarked, "God and family are what matter most. The rest is just stuff."

Supplication

With gratitude, I undeservedly
Accept the sacrifice You made for me.
At times I deviate, again am lost.
Forgetting my salvation's wretched cost.
I stray and am distracted from my task.
Again I seek Your peace; once more, I ask:
That You would draw me near, reset my course;
Be all I think and do and say—my Source.
Renew, refresh, regenerate my heart,
Assign my work, equip me for my part:
A conduit for You to those I know.
Your kingdom's grace and mercy to them show:
To lift them from despair and agony,
That by Your stripes, they too, may be made free!

Your Reflections

1. Describe the story of your faith journey—how did it begin and progress throughout your life?

2. In what ways have you found yourself distracted or misled, straying from the Way throughout your life?

3. Have you returned, and if so, what happened to cause your return? If not, what are some reasons holding you back?

4. What books, music, or other resources in your life have lured your thinking in the wrong direction, and what do you want to do about it?

5. What has been your experience of being thought a fool for the sake of the gospel?

6. How has your declining health impacted your relationship with God? With others?

7. What has been your experience of shifting your focus away from yourself and onto God?

8. How would you describe your own experience of being in the world, yet not of it?

9. What is your sense of your inner spirit growing even as your outer shell withers?

10. *Prayer:* Write out your thoughts to God concerning your meandering path on the way to your Heavenly home. Give thanks to Him for shepherding you.

Chapter Six

The Inner Circle

People draw near to help prepare us for our homegoing.

How does our impending departure affect them, and how do they impact us?

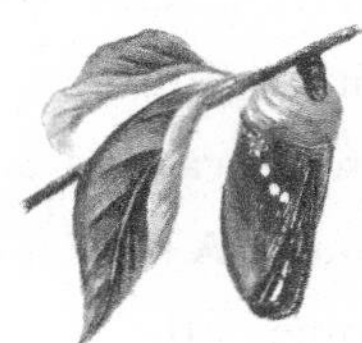

We can always tell when it's time to leave a party. Even if we've had a great time, our attention begins to drift away from what once held our interest and still holds everyone else's rapt attention. They are chatting animatedly, fully engaged, and we are smiling and nodding as we pretend interest in small talk. We look for that gap in the conversation where we can gracefully make closure to signal our exit.

"It was wonderful to see you!"

"Let's do this again soon!"

The party may still be in full swing with new revelers arriving while others dance, tell jokes, or play games. Some have already slipped out quietly. Some have gestured broadly while calling out a booming salutation to everyone within earshot. Threading our way to the door, we see that some are too absorbed to notice our approaching departure, still others make eye contact and wave from across the room. Those who know us more intimately walk us to the door, perhaps even to the car for the long, Midwest goodbye. We know that if the tables were turned, we would want to be by their side for as long as we could, too. Away from the din indoors and out into the fresh air, we are relieved to be free, accompanied only by those with whom we can be ourselves. It's not that the party was boring or that anyone there was offensive. It's just that it's time to leave. We need rest and quiet, and the loud chaos, jovial though it was, is now grating to our souls, while we yearn for tranquility.

I am still at the party right now. It's been a good one, and I've gotten to make so many friends and enjoy so much, but it's about time to go. I've begun to see the waves from across the room, and some have approached to send me off with sweet tokens of kindness: flowers, notes, home visits, texts or calls, meals, care boxes, treat bags, beautiful handmade arts, chocolates, and more. A smaller cadre has gathered with me at the door. Interestingly, some of the ones who are walking me to the door are newer friends, while older ones have made the wave across the room. It isn't disconcerting in the slightest. Rather, it has meant that every day is novel and full of surprises as friends emerge from the most unexpected places and times. It is more clear than ever which friendships and family connections are the strongest, and I have no idea why. Kurt Vonnegut, in his 1963 novel, *The Cat's Cradle*, has an especially creative way of explaining this phenomenon.[9]

Vonnegut describes the two groups of people to which we belong. He devised the term "karass," referring to a network of people that are linked together to fulfill the will of God. These people do not intentionally form bonds with each other and may not even know each other, but they always instantly and warmly recognize one another as belonging to the same karass. A "granfalloon," on the other hand, is an intentional but meaningless collection of people. A granfalloon is a false karass. He explains that people come together under a hollow title that unites them superficially but try as they might, there are no real bonds forged in such a superfluous gathering. Some examples are fraternities and sororities, civic clubs and organizations, and academic graduating classes. Such associations fill our time with busywork and appear to be significant. They may accomplish service projects together or strive for a good cause, but little of eternally valuable consequence results from their union.

While Vonnegut's constructs here are fictitious, the descriptions aptly match our experience. Applied to our party scenario, we will never find our granfalloon partners walking us to the door. Our karass brothers and sisters emerge strong, supporting our every step until we roll away from the curb. This is our inner circle, and it will look different for everyone. Some of us have large families while others have none, some are extroverts with a large group of friends while others are introverts who have one or two loyal friends. Many factors contribute to the formation of our inner circle; they vary in size. My hospice team of Beth, Casie, and Tom share that they have seen every conceivable kind of configuration. It is not uncommon for people to spend their final days and weeks with no companions at all, and the hospice team itself becomes the inner circle.

[The people in my inner circle] are nothing less than God's divinely appointed agents.

There is no more difficult writing task than to describe my inner circle and what it has meant to me. It is difficult because there is no way to express how indispensable each of them has been. They are nothing less than God's divinely appointed agents. I know He is near in ways described earlier, but He is also near in that He has provided people who know just what to say, what to do, and how to provide much needed encouragement. They uplift without condescension, help without making me feel they're doing me a big favor, and support while acting as if it is their privilege. I count myself blessed many times over by these family members and friends, no less than the examples of friendship and family in the Bible. I think about the loyal friends David and Jonathan, who loved each other with such brotherly affection. Ruth's devotion to Naomi is another such example of beautiful steadfastness, as is Boaz's integrity. If you do not know the Biblical accounts of these people, it is worth picking up your Bible and taking the time to learn what loyalty really looks like.

My people are no different than these. I find myself surrounded by such incredibly constant and faithful friends and family, and I am overwhelmed with gratitude. They express support in various ways including frequent check-in texts, calls, in-home visits, invitations to coffee or lunch, making a huge bag of homemade treats for our family road trip, help with this writing project, and help with necessary tasks of living that I cannot always perform. There is no way I can adequately capture how thankful I am for this inner circle, these people whose involvement in my life at this hard time have demonstrated love in action. They help in different ways.

Proverbs 27:9 brings to mind those cheerful ones who give honest, helpful suggestions. It reads: "Perfume and incense bring joy to the heart, and the pleasantness of a friend springs from their heartfelt advice." They inquire about nutrition, suggest ways to stay comfortable, and give practical counsel. My hospice nurse, Beth, is a great example of this. She visits weekly and gives useful guidance. When I was a cancer patient under Dr. Zhang's care, I also had a Nurse Navigator, Monica. I could not have managed without her. From the moment she got involved with my case, she provided every kind of help. When you've just lost twelve inches of your colon, let's just say you need lots of advice. When you've been to the doctor and you think you heard everything he said, but then you get home and realize you've forgotten half of it, you need a Monica. I could call or text her at any time, and she had access to the doctor's notes. Even now that I am no longer under an oncologist's care, she still checks in, and I will always be thankful for her humor, her expertise, and her brown cow recipe.

Even smaller is the ring who, in especially hard circumstances, have set their own needs aside to care for me, sitting long hours on the hard chair next to mine during infusions. Their obedience to 1 Corinthians 10:24 has been steadfast: "Let no one seek his own good, but the good of his neighbor." I could substitute the word "neighbor" with wife, mom, cousin, or friend. Eric was my most frequent companion by the chemo chair. Erica popped in frequently to check on me. Logan and his wife Jill accompanied for some doctor visits and chemo chair days as well. Some good friends and family members stepped in for these too, giving my immediate family a break. My mother was always close at hand to visit afterward, eager to help. Church friends and my sister-in-law brought meals on days there was no way we were in shape to cook. What selflessness each of these exhibited.

Those who simply offer companionship and pleasant company bring to life Psalm 133: "How good and pleasant it is when God's people live together in unity!" At times, there are those few who will engage in theological discussion where we seek to get to the heart of a spiritual truth or scriptural passage, embodying Proverbs 27:17, "As iron sharpens iron, so one person sharpens another." These are the people who give of their time to visit, and we don't even have to talk about cancer. These people continue to bless with their sense of humor, candor, and friendship. I treasure the afternoon teas, the late night texts, the prayer time, the nail appointments, the trips to stay here with us for a few days. These are the inner rings forming the circle who will carry us homeward.

The innermost ring of a dying person's circle are the immediate caregivers, close family members or friends who do the hard work no one else does or sees. They know the details no one else knows. I have not yet reached a point of needing this kind of care, and I'm not looking forward to it, either. Who wants to put loved ones through helping with toileting, dressing, and hygiene? When we get to the stage of adult diapers, I shudder to think of my husband or grown kids helping. I hope to avoid having family members do this, but I don't know if that will be possible. Such arrangements are common and necessary in some cases, and I am admittedly squeamish about it. However, I know not to fight it.

The innermost ring of a dying person's circle are the immediate caregivers, close family members or friends who do the hard work no one else does or sees.

Tom, Casie, and Beth have become part of that innermost ring, as hospice workers who intimately know the details of my case and who will journey with us to the end. Because I have enrolled in hospice early, our conversations are different than ones they often have with patients, who are closer to death than I (presumably) am. This has afforded time for me to ask them about their work, which I find fascinating. That people would choose a career devoted to shepherding others to the gate is curious, and I have found that these unique people have a special calling. They have a wealth of experience in companioning the dying, that final act of our existence that few witness. They have seen every conceivable family scenario, every socio-economic level, and nearly every type of death ranging from agonizing to peaceful to euphoric.

Because dying involves everyone in the innermost circle, not just the person dying, I asked Tom, Casie, and Beth what they have noticed about these relationships. Here is a summary of their answers.

What patient behaviors make end-of-life care hard on family and caregivers?

- When family members and the patient are not in agreement on being hospice-oriented, everything is harder.
- Some find it hard to accept that the family member is dying, which creates tension and difficulty for the patient.
- At times, families will push their agenda over the patient's well-being, and patients do not always advocate for themselves, going along with the family instead. It would be better for the patient if the focus were kept on his/her needs first.
- When patients try to maintain independence instead of accepting help, fighting the process, it can become a stressful environment. When anger is misplaced in the form of trying to control what's happening, caregivers can be frustrated.

What are some things the dying can do to lessen the burden on family and caregivers?

- Ask for help, but still do what we can do.
- Take the hospice team's suggestions.
- Accept that we now have limitations. We cannot do what we were once able to do for ourselves, and we are better off to embrace this.
- Do all we can to be at peace in our relationships with others; say what needs to be said.
- Accept that it is okay to die.

In one's last months and weeks of life, relationship issues often surface. Tom, Casie, and Beth have witnessed and often mediated cases where there was so much discord that their patients' well-being was compromised. This is a serious crunch-time for families who must come together for the good of the one who is dying, and if there is disharmony, it must be dealt with. For the patients themselves, reflection time afforded by days of being bedridden often brings regrets, or in some cases, epiphanies, or both. For my father-in-law, Nolan, it was both.

He had worked in the grocery business since the 1940s after his return home from Germany after World War II. He wasted no time marrying his girl, Betty, and over the next twenty years, four sons were born. Nolan loved the grocery business, managing and then owning several of them, mostly in small towns. First to arrive each day and last to leave, he was a business owner who did not entrust many details to others, which meant that while he was married to Betty, the grocery store was a bit of a rival spouse. Fortunately, Betty was supportive of Nolan's work and helped him as much as she could in between raising four boys and caring for their home. When Eric and I began dating, it was immediately clear that his parents were of a different generation than my own. My parents had married young and were baby boomers maturing during the sixties with Motown tunes or Janis Joplin on eight-track tapes blasting over the speakers as they worked around the house in their bell-bottomed jeans. Mom made dinner every night and served it herself onto our plates, dishing up comfort food directly from the pans in which it was cooked. Dad ate his in front of the TV while I ate at the kitchen table and mom ate at the countertop pull-out. It was a fun, functional family, but it functioned differently than Eric's.

The first time I went to Eric's house for dinner, I was amazed at the way Betty had prepared the table. She routinely used china dishes and set the table formally every night. Main courses and side dishes were served from platters and patterned bowls. Small crystal saucers held a variety of relishes, and dessert usually followed the meal of meat, potatoes, salad, and vegetable. Grace was said before the food was served, and it was always served family style. This meant that everyone actually gathered at the table together, and there was conversation about the day's business. After I had come around for a while, I noticed the music in the background was usually some classic country artist like Jim Reeves or Loretta Lynn. The values were essentially the same in our homes, but the style of doing things was different, and I came to understand that this was because his parents were of the Greatest Generation, ones who were born before the Great Depression and lived through World War II. Eric's oldest brother, born in the mid-1940s, was close in age to my parents. Eric and I were close in age, but our homes were culturally different because of the gap in our parents' ages.

He wasted no time marrying his girl, Betty, and over the next twenty years, four sons were born.

Despite the differences, I still enjoyed being with Eric's family. The dinnertime conversations were lively and fun, and the banter between them was surprising to me. Nolan's ways spoke volumes of his generation's understanding about gender roles without saying a word. This is not to say he was an overbearing Archie Bunker; he was anything but. Kind, quiet, and dry-witted, he strove to get along with everyone. He simply lived in a way typical of those born in his era. The woman ran the home, and the man worked outside it. The simple, traditional arrangement was taken for granted. His dinner was served at six every evening, and afterward, he retired to the living room while Betty did the dishes. There is no need to inflate the number of words written on women's rights in today's culture; they are abundantly covered. On his own, Nolan revisited the topic years later from his nursing home room.

His years as a widower did not change his lifestyle much, except he had to do his laundry, and his dinner was not the magnificent affair it had once been. He continued his work at the grocery store just as always, arriving early, departing late, eating meals at noon and six, and sleeping in his recliner until he could start again. This was the life he liked, and he held onto it as long as possible, beyond the point of being safely advisable. He had developed an autoimmune disease, myocitis, which caused his muscle tissue to deteriorate starting with the large muscles such as thighs, abdominals, and arms, eventually working its way down to smaller muscles that controlled fine motor movement. The trajectory in myocitis is that the patient gradually loses mobility in every way, eventually being motionless. It does not affect cognitive capacity but does imprison the patient inside his own body much like ALS.

Nolan was able to cope with this condition for several years by using special equipment such as a lift van, walker, stair chair, lift chair, special silverware, and a few other assists. Striving hard to maintain his work routine, he had employees stationed at various points to help him in and out of his stair chair and into his office chair, and his sons were always nearby to help him at home when needed. There came a time, though, when he was hospitalized for a UTI, and the doctors recognized the danger he was in as a fall risk. He was not released to go home but was instead sent to a nursing home and rehabilitation center. This was not at all to his liking, but he was far beyond the point of his routine being smoothly achievable. Several small catastrophes had occurred already, and while he disliked this new arrangement, it was a relief to family who could no longer manage his care.

He skipped the small talk and disclosed what was on his mind: his conscience.

Even though he had faithful daily visitors, there were now many quiet hours to reflect upon his life. Everyone who knew Nolan knew that he was honest, hard-working, and trustworthy. He had maintained good relationships with his sons and their wives, and the grandchildren adored him. He also had a wonderful lady friend who had been his faithful companion for many years, and they had enjoyed many good times together that Nolan was missing so wistfully. It could be assumed that his reflections would be all positive ones, looking back on years well-spent, enjoying his success at being a good provider for his family, and knowing his solid reputation in the community. I would never have known otherwise except for one evening when I popped in for a visit with him, alone. He was uncharacteristically quiet, and the TV was off. I tried to engage him in conversation, and he quickly skipped the small talk and disclosed what was on his mind: his conscience. Nolan, in honest humility, had looked in the mirror and had not liked the reflection.

He began to tearfully describe the early years he and Betty were married, where she worked all day at his store, took care of house and the yard, raised the boys, cooked and cleaned up dinner, then sat on the kitchen floor making signs in her immaculate script for his grocery store windows back in the days when it had to be done with enormous sheets of white paper and wide markers. He recalled coming home to a dinner she had prepared, then leaving the table for hours of TV in his recliner while her workday continued until bedtime. He could have tried justifying this with the generous gifts he had given her, but he did not.

He recalled the holidays and birthdays she always worked so hard to make festive and special with minimal help from him. Again, he did not attempt to defend himself by saying he provided the income, or was too busy. His honest recollection was that Betty had been the one who worked so hard to make sure the family would have wonderful holiday memories. No one talked about these things. That's just the way it was. Nolan never made chauvinist remarks, but he was now faced with the way he had lived, letting Betty do the majority of the work around the home and yard as well as managing the kids, and he was not proud. No one in his family held resentment toward him; he was responsible and hard-working. Even so, he was not pleased with himself. As I listened, another subject emerged.

"I don't know how to say it. I guess it's that they are precious. They are precious to me."

Nolan had become a favorite at the nursing home. The aides were all friendly with him, and he grew quite attached to them. They were by default a part of his inner circle. Most of these aides were of varied ethnic origins different than his, and his previous experience with people of other ethnicities had been limited. Now he depended on them for everything. Still tearful, he described the work they dutifully and cheerfully did on his behalf. He talked about their children and families, and some of the problems they had related to him. Then he began to talk about what they had meant to him. After describing them and their admirable qualities he concluded his speech, saying that he never realized how alike all people were, with the same problems and concerns. At last, he said, "I don't know how to say it. I guess it's that they are precious. They are precious to me." He was overwhelmed with gratitude for these nurses' aides who had become so important to him, and he cared about each of them individually. While he disliked being stuck at the nursing home, he loved those who took such good care of him.

After his soul was unburdened, he slipped into serene sleep. He had been a believer all these years, long ago having been justified by Christ's atoning death and resurrection. Nolan's unsettled emotions were the stirrings of a Christian whose repentant heart needed the restorative work of Christ, sanctifying him through it to prepare him for Heaven. Mingled with gratitude as well, his light shone brightly even though he was unaware of it himself.

Not more than a year later, he was in the hospital again. It was yet another UTI, and his body was becoming resistant to the antibiotics. Nolan motioned me to his bedside, and with a suspicious twinkle in his eye, he declared with finality, "I'm going home!" At first, I thought he was delirious as he had sometimes been with previous UTIs, referring to his house that had been vacant for four years. He had longed to go back to his house, openly yearning for more time to enjoy life with his family, his special companion, and his business. But I was puzzled—he seemed too clear-eyed and certain to be delusional. I responded to him with a tentative smile, not knowing what to say. Hours later, it struck me: he was telling me that his death was near, that he was going to his Heavenly home. I regret that it took me so long to realize it, and I never had the chance to ask him to elaborate, or to explain how he knew his time was near. Eric and his brothers understood the situation the doctor presented, and they consented to hospice. Nolan was soon transported to Harry Hynes Hospice, and I was a little taken aback to discover he inhabited the very room my own father had died in a few years before.

He slept through most of the next few days as family visited, his breathing progressively more labored into the Cheyne-Stokes breathing I had seen with my own father. Eric's oldest brother and his wife, as well as Logan and Jill, had stood at Nolan's bedside one afternoon. They observed his breathing pattern, its tempo slowing. All at once, he was bright-eyed, looking to his left. He was looking through Jill and Logan who were standing by, fixed intently on something no one else could see. His eyes tracked across the horizon before closing again, his countenance peacefully at rest. No one present could have doubted that he was welcomed into his Heavenly home just as he had predicted a few days before. His conscience was clear, he was at peace with all who knew him, and now he would enjoy the company of his Savior and of those who had gone before. Both Betty and Nolan were much loved and are missed, and their family will be glad for the day of our reunion in Heaven.

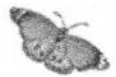

The Four Things That Matter Most: A Book About Living, by author Ira Byock, M.D., who has worked more than twenty-five years in hospice and palliative care came highly recommended to me. True to its reputation, it was hard to put down. Byock shares the simple idea that taking care of our relationships and bringing closure to old wounds can be done by expressing four things:

> *Please forgive me.*
> *I forgive you.*
> *Thank you.*
> *I love you.*[10]

We all have histories, lives that were lived before we gained much wisdom or sound judgment. We have all done and said things that need to be made right. Denial, blaming, grudges, and excuse-making only widen the chasm between ourselves and the other person(s). Deep down we know this, but even thinking back to these events causes the buried emotions to reach up from the crypt, entrapping us and disabling our efforts to make amends. Even when we know the fault isn't ours, we want closure. We want to know we did everything we could to leave the world and everyone in it free from any toxicity that memories of us may trigger.

Byock's book takes the hard task and breaks it into words that are feasible for anyone, and the effects are staggeringly powerful. He tells story after story of relationships being restored and renewed, with some at the very least being patched together acceptably. There are heart-wrenching accounts of people forgiving abusers, expressing love toward toxic, hateful parents, all making amends of formerly ruinous, broken filial bonds. This is not to say that every relationship was renewed. But poisonous loose ends left uncauterized over decades were treated and sealed in satisfactory results for all parties, and nearly always, the words were reciprocated. Even if not, there is rest in knowing we did all we could do. Romans 12:18 confirms, "If possible, so far as it depends on you, live peaceably with all." What difficulties remain are not ours to own.

He acknowledges that not all families say Byock's "Four Things" in the same way. In one case, Byock describes a father-son relationship as the father was in his final weeks. A farm family of German heritage and Lutheran upbringing, they had close, loyal relationships but were not overtly demonstrative either physically or verbally. Still father and son loved one another and desired to spend time together. The father's care had become too difficult for his wife, and she had placed him in a nursing home. There, the son came to visit, gradually taking part in his father's physical care. Unaccustomed to such personal contact, the son began by taking over his father's shaving routine, using warm towels and facial massage. Eventually taking over many of the other aspects of his care, the son wordlessly demonstrating love for his father, and the father's acceptance of his son's help showed wordless reciprocation to his son. Through this intimate shaving ritual that expanded to feeding, toileting, and dressing, the "Four Things" were addressed without saying the words out loud.

Tom, Casie, and Beth would advise the same: forgive, accept apologies, apologize, do what we can to mend relationships. Broken, fractious relationships make for difficult passages for the dying and for our families. When a family member's death, or our own death approaches, it is a time to let go of old hurts and release grudges we have nursed over the years. It is time to let the balm of these verses from God's word sink into our souls and penetrate each wound:

> Be kind to one another, tenderhearted, forgiving one another, as God in Christ forgave you. (Ephesians 4:32)
>
> . . . bearing with one another, and forgiving each other, whoever has a complaint against anyone; just as the Lord forgave you, so you also must forgive. Beyond all these things put on love, which is the perfect bond of unity. (Colossians 3:13,14)
>
> Therefore, accept one another, just as Christ also accepted us to the glory of God. (Romans 15:7)
>
> Gracious words are like a honeycomb, sweetness to the soul and health to the body. (Proverbs 16:24)
>
> A new commandment I give to you, that you love one another: just as I have loved you, you also are to love one another. (John 13:34)
>
> If we confess our sins, He is faithful and just to forgive us our sins and to cleanse us from all unrighteousness. (1 John 1:9)

And once more,

> If possible, so far as it depends on you, live peaceably with all. (Romans 12:18)

There is nothing to lose except pride in accepting these consoling words that call us to peacemaking. We lose pride not in the sense of losing our dignity, but in the sense of losing the stubbornness of a child who clings to wanting her own way. Pride is likely what led us into these conflicts to begin with and courageously laying it down is the only way out. It feels like an act of weakness to give in but is quite the opposite. Think of examples you've seen where people have sacrificed their pride for a greater good. It is always an act of strength and valor, and those who can do it are remembered in a positive light.

Tom, Casie, and Beth further advise patients to let go of what we can no longer do and allow others to help us. This is easy to understand when applied to other people. When we apply the advice to ourselves, it is much harder. Most of us do not like being the recipient of others' help. We would rather do the helping. Yet we have already seen that all things are made beautiful in their time. There is a time to help and a time to accept help. We all have our reasons for resisting this seemingly simple turn of events. For me, it is hard. Why?

Think of examples you've seen where people have sacrificed their pride for a greater good. It is always an act of strength and valor.

I have been the sick one, getting all the attention, the cards and flowers and gifts. All the time to relax at home. All the calls and texts and prayers. In the background, quietly toiling, is my husband. He has sacrificed days off hauling me to appointments, sitting in crowded, fluorescent-lit rooms hostage to *The View* on wall-mounted televisions when he could be golfing. Many beautiful days when we might have taken our kayaks to the lake or worked in our flower beds, he now spent watching poison slowly drip into my veins.

At home, the imbalance continues. Our household chores once functioned well for us both. Since my energy has decreased, I've let go of a few responsibilities, and while I have kept up with many things like cooking and laundry and maintenance cleaning, this won't last forever, and he will have to take these over, too. He now does more cleanup after meals, as I am often tired after cooking. He takes care of all the yard chores, the cat's litterbox and feeding, and carrying anything that needs lifting. When we were younger, it wasn't unusual for him to come home from work and discover that I had moved all the furniture or spent the whole day working in the flowerbeds. Now, he often must carry the laundry basket upstairs and get the groceries hauled in. He quietly absorbs these changes without complaint.

This is what ending, losing, and letting go looks and feels like.

These are small changes but taken together they are not. I know that he will soon assume responsibility for their entirety. He can do the work, but that isn't the problem. I liked carrying my weight. I liked the balance of work in our home, and I felt that my contributions to the running of our household had value.

This is what ending, losing, and letting go looks and feels like. It's more than just words on a paper. In our last months, weeks, and days of life, we must recognize we no longer bring value to our families in terms of what we can do for them, or how we can offset the labors that must be performed. In fact, we now necessitate others' labors, and that is abhorrent to us. It is then that we must remember that these downward steps denoting our progressing condition are normal. Expect them.

This happens to everyone, and it just happens to be our turn. It gives rest for us to remember that our lives are changing, but the love of God will not. 1 John 4:16 declares,

> So we have come to know and to believe the love that God has for us. God is love, and whoever abides in love abides in God, and God abides in him.

To trust God, accept change, and be gracious to those near us is now our new role. We cannot do the heavy lifting, but we can be uplifting encouragers.

Accepting that our illness is creating work for others is not easy, but to refuse help is to remain prideful, and we only make the situation harder by getting in the way and interfering with people who are better equipped. When we are too fragile to be helpful, we are cumbersome if we try to insist on doing things our way. There is a time to accept help. We are wise to know when that time has come, and to relax into it, knowing we would want to help them if roles were reversed.

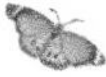

In chapter four, I mentioned Gerry and Aggie. Early in their marriage, no one could have guessed the scenario that developed in its final years. His athleticism had always featured prominently. Aggie recalls that they often spent four or five nights each week at a ballfield either watching or playing. While she might have preferred spending their together time elsewhere, she recognized what a great guy she had and resolved to make the best of it. They played softball, watched live sports, watched televised sports, and talked about sports.

Aggie shares the story of their marriage beautifully, and she is beautiful woman herself. Nearly seventy, her figure is as trim as any sixteen-year-old, and her blonde hair is long and fashionably curled back. She may be small, but she is strong and agile, and radiates energy. Their back yard is a maze of walkways, bridges, flower beds, trellises, and rocks, most of it her doing. Part of her fitness could be attributed to her health-conscious cooking. She worked hard to maintain good nutrition for herself and Gerry, making meals from scratch, including her homemade bread.

It came as a shock to all who knew them when Gerry was diagnosed with ALS in 2013. While they had an army of friends and family, and a church family as well, Aggie was the main caregiver for Gerry, who felt most comfortable in her capable hands. Fit as she was, Gerry was a big man, and at two hundred-plus pounds, she had her hands full. He sometimes fell, needing the fire department to come to their rescue. He once fell onto Aggie, who was able to brace herself on a door frame and safely lower the two of them to the floor, avoiding the serious injury that doubtless would have happened were it not for her breaking the fall.

As Gerry's health declined, he graduated from hanging on to doorways and furniture, to using a walker, to eventually spending his last two-and-a-half years in his lift chair.

Aggie was aware something was wrong before Gerry was. She noticed a strangeness in his gait, where his feet seemed to flop instead of walk with controlled steps. And then there were instances where he would fall while running the bases, something that had never happened before. Gerry had been a superb athlete, so Aggie's concerns grew as she witnessed the gradual loss of coordination.

The diagnosis eventually came, but for a while it was suspected that he could have Lyme disease, and there was hope that he might be able to find an effective treatment. The situation progressed, though, and over the next two-and-a-half years, resulted in his being unable to care for even the most routine habits of personal care, such as grooming, dressing, and toileting. Aggie took care of it all and was honored to do it. With the help of the fire department, she moved their living quarters to the basement so that Gerry would be safe if there were a tornado, and accommodations were added to create a way of escape in case of fire. She was able to cook in the basement as well, so they truly were constant companions. She is a licensed massage therapist as well as having a few other income streams that were easily operated from home, so there was seldom a reason to leave him, and if she did need to run an errand, she had someone look after him for a few minutes.

As Aggie spoke so reverently of her husband, I was struck by her resourcefulness and her faith, and with the sense that even though they had friends, family, and church, ALS was something the two of them really had to deal with on their own. Church friends came frequently at first and prayed with them, which brought a great deal of encouragement and comfort. It became clear that Gerry wasn't getting better, though, and the church friends who had come at first slowly trickled away. Aggie does not make assumptions as to why this happened. The illness was prolonged, people have their own lives, and she prefers not to worry about why, focusing instead on gratitude for those who faithfully brought meals and were consistently kind and thoughtful.

While a support system would have been helpful, Aggie was so consumed with working and taking care of Gerry and running the household, though, that she had little time to worry about that. Aggie described how his skin had begun to break down due to being in his lift chair twenty-four hours a day. He slept in it because of the difficulty of getting in and out of bed and finding ways to get comfortable. To prevent pressure ulcers from forming, she developed a skin care routine for him and was pleased that throughout this whole time, he was spared the discomfort of that added misery. It is worthwhile to detail what she did, should others benefit from her discovery.

Gerry's skin care routine involved keeping him clean and dry and using skin cream on him, but she also had a tool called DermaWand®,[11] which aestheticians use in facial massages to improve skin tone. This little device worked wonders, stimulating his skin in areas where it had begun to redden, the first sign of an ulcer. The online advertisement for the DermaWand® reads,

> Dramatically younger-looking skin in just three minutes a day. All the benefits of professional radio frequency technology, DermaWand® reduces the appearance of wrinkles and pores, tightens aging skin all in the comfort of your own home.

It also does a lot more, as Aggie discovered, that went unadvertised. Gerry never had a single pressure ulcer.

Even though his care was cumbersome and physically demanding, Aggie had nothing but praise for Gerry and his attitude. Instead, her lament was that he could not even so much as remove a tickling stray hair or scratch an itch, annoying sensations that are easily relieved for the rest of us who take for granted our ability to do so. For the immobile, those sensations are no small thing; they are exasperating. Aggie was by Gerry's side for these seemingly small needs as well as the big ones. She did everything possible to keep him comfortable, to keep his skin healthy, keep him fed, keep him clean, and keep him company. Often, they slept holding hands, his chair beside the bed or by the sofa.

Often they slept holding hands, his chair beside the bed or by the sofa.

His care, given willingly and lovingly, had demanded much from her. Over a Memorial Day weekend, Aggie had been treated in the hospital for exhaustion. She had also been to the doctor to treat pain in her thoracic area, an injury sustained in doing the physical work of caring for him. She still has so much gratitude for the nurses and physical therapists that were able to help some, but it wasn't enough to offset the toll on her own body. A month later, on June 28, Gerry passed away. It happened when the doorbell rang and Aggie went up to take a delivery, visiting for a few minutes with the woman who had rung. Returning to the basement, she found Gerry sitting in his chair with a peaceful expression on his face, his spirit having flown.

The two of them had never discussed death. Gerry had behaved as if he believed that one day he would get up out of his chair and walk again, and they simply never had a conversation about what might happen otherwise. Aggie still is not sure what happened in those minutes while she was upstairs. There had been no sign of anything abnormal. He had eaten a huge breakfast that morning and was watching his favorite TV program when she ran upstairs. The breathing device Gerry used was still functional, but she found him resting peacefully without his mouth pressed against it. She trusts that God knows, and that is enough.

Exhausted and now brokenhearted as well, she had done everything possible to make Gerry's life relaxed and peaceful, and he had done everything he could to express gratitude for her work with consistent kindness. His behavior during these physical and emotional struggles did not falter. He had always been the kind of man who forgave easily and could see all perspectives in a conflict. He sought to be at peace with others always, even in the most difficult circumstances. Even when he was betrayed.

Gerry worked with unmatched fidelity for his employer. He was loyal to the company and believed in its products, working steadfastly to promote growth in the business and success in its clients. He had every reason to believe he was valued by those in the top tier of the organization, considering most of them close friends, even brothers. When Gerry disclosed his health condition to these friends and co-workers, he was immediately dismissed. There was no compensation, and worse, there were no words of sorrow or encouragement. He was simply discarded with harsh, casual disregard. What a painful gut-punch to both Gerry and Aggie, whose trust in these duplicitous "friends" now lay in ruins amid the most unfair of circumstances. Gerry could have chosen any number of responses. What he chose was forgiveness. The man whose body deteriorated more each day had an already—strong spirit that grew more gallant with each hardship. He forgave those who did not visit as one might expect, too. In sum, Gerry's Christ-centered character was valiant. It was Aggie's good pleasure to serve him well.

While she had a little help, she could have used much more. Hospice could have provided so much more support, securing that reliable inner circle that both needed. Hospice provides volunteers, home health aides, social workers, nurses, and chaplains. While friends and family are important, these other hands-on resources are critical in mitigating caregiver fatigue, which Aggie certainly experienced. For hospice to be secured, though, there must be a realization that death is, at the very least, a possibility. In their case, neither wanted to give up hope.

Gerry's death has been life-changing for Aggie. She finds solace in reading God's word, and her faith has strengthened. She recalls the day Gerry received the phone call terminating his employment, on her birthday. She relives a moment where she stood at the window wondering what it would be like to care for someone with a terminal illness and suddenly have no income. There were no savings, nothing to fall back on. They had mortgage payments on two homes—one in Florida and their current Kansas home, car payments, and some credit card debt. Aggie describes the situation like Jesus feeding the crowd with only a few loaves and fishes. Not once did they go hungry, and they continued to live in their home, where she still resides. She says, "Somehow God worked a miracle, and I was able to care for him and provide enough income to keep us afloat. Yes, some things were carved out. A lot of things. And a few things were lost, but we had everything we needed." She had placed her trust and faith in God, saying to Him, "I don't know what this is going to look like, but You do." And He did.

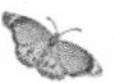

Aggie's story is heartbreaking. I suspect it is uncommon to find two people in such circumstances whose most pressing concern is each other instead of self. However, I don't think stories of exhausted caregivers are rare. Caregivers, widows, and widowers are all around us, each with a story that needs to be shared, and each with needs that the church has been charged to meet. We must remember that our busy lives will resume after the funeral dinner dishes have been cleared, but the widow(er)'s will not. James 1:27 instructs, "Religion that is pure and undefiled before God the father is this: to visit orphans and widows in their affliction . . . " Thankfully, many churches now provide groups called Grief Share, where those who have lost someone can process their grief together and find solace in knowing they are not alone in enduring it. This is a step in the right direction, to "visit widows in their affliction," although there is no substitute for being present and listening well.

Hospice could have provided so much more support, securing that reliable inner circle that both needed.

In the first chapter, I wrote about how this happened with my mother. I could not grieve for her. No one could carry the grief for her; it must be borne alone, and no one can fill the void. In mom's case, church family did check in on her, as did neighbors and family. I visited her every evening for quite a while. Dad had done everything possible to have his affairs in order, but still, her inner life was in disarray for a few years. For widow(er)s, the work of grieving a spouse is a lonely experience no matter how much others want to help. One thing Dad did was to encourage me in keeping mom's life alive and interesting. He asked me not to just look in on her regularly, but to give her things to look forward to. I am not sure I would have thought of this on my own, and it was good advice.

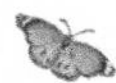

Ultimately, once we are gone, we cannot help the grieving. Beyond having our legal affairs in order and suggesting that family keep the momentum of family life going, this is one of those items on the "Letting Go" list. We are not indispensable, and people will figure out what to do when we are gone. Tom and Casie, as well as other friends, have also suggested writing letters, making voice recordings, and taking pictures and videos to preserve relationship memories. The time comes, though, that we are gone, and our inner circle disbands. It is broken by our departure. The circle dissipates, and new patterns and ways of living will emerge.

One last thing we can do for our spouse and/or closest loved ones is pray for them, that their lives will be full of meaningful activity, blessing, and fulfillment. That God will draw near to them and comfort them, giving them peace. That an inner circle will form around them, supporting and nurturing them in our absence. We can pray this Scripture over them: "And the peace of God, which surpasses all understanding, will guard your hearts and your minds in Christ Jesus" (Philippians 4:7).

Your Reflections

1. Who did you think would be in your inner circle, and how has that compared to the actual?

2. What do these people do that you are especially thankful for, and in what ways do you let them know of your gratitude?

3. Who do you need to say the "Four Things" to, and how might you go about doing this? Who could help you prepare to do it?

4. What does your long look in the mirror reveal, and what needs repentance and forgiveness before you approach others with the "Four Things"?

5. Anticipate possible responses you might receive and how you want to be sure you respond.

6. If you have a spouse/significant other, what do you anticipate will be the most difficult for them when you have passed?

7. What are some small provisions you could make now to ease their time later on (writing a letter, putting together a folder with important information, etc.)?

8. What will be especially hard for you to accept when you must let a caregiver do things for you, and what do you want to remember from this chapter about that?

9. If you are a church attender, who might you talk to about keeping in touch with your spouse/significant other to keep him/her involved and active?

10. Write out your prayer for your inner circle. What do you want to ask God to do for each of them after you have passed on? Give thanks for each of them, as they are His gifts to you.

Chapter Seven

Life in the Slow Lane

Deceleration doesn't have to be depressing.

What roses have we neglected to smell in our busier phase of life?

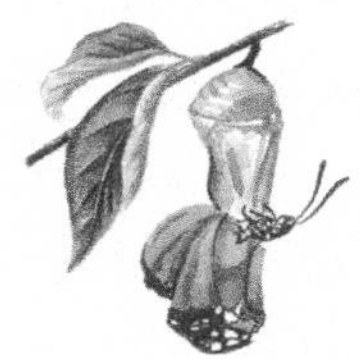

"**The word of the day** is energy conservation," Beth sweetly scolded as she left today. She's telling me to slow down. To recognize there is less energy available, so spend it carefully. What does a full day look like when you're no longer working, not capable of putting in a full day of labor at home either, but still alive enough to be awake and aware, with surges of activity between rests? I was curious about this, wondering if everyone in my shoes walked the same way throughout a day, so I asked my friend Angela, the music teacher with late stage cancer I mentioned in chapter four. She described her day as getting up around 7:30 a.m., showering and doing personal maintenance, then having breakfast. She rests for a while, then spends the day doing things that feed her soul. She reads her Bible, listens to music, and does small chores around her home that don't require a lot of energy. Yep. That's about what my day looks like. An observer might be quickly bored. A day like this doesn't look like much. How deceiving appearances can be!

There is no rule book stating how we are supposed to spend our time when we don't have much of it left. There wasn't a rule book before, either, but it was much easier to move through a day when everyone around me was doing about the same thing at the same pace. I heard once that human life, as designed by the Creator, moves at about three miles per hour. That's the average walking pace, and when most transport was on foot, most moved together at that comfortable rate. Moving in sync with one's peers is something we take for granted until we are sick. Recall a time when you had to call in sick to work, and when you returned, life had gone on without you. It took a bit to get your bearings and find your way back into the flow. Now, our walking pace may be about the same, but life moves much faster than ever before, faster than most of us short-timers would prefer. To be out of the flow is to become isolated, and for some, this is the hardest part of being ill.

Competitive cycling was Eric's hobby for a while. He was one of those people you see on the roadside in spandex and helmets, wearing a camel pack canteen and shoes that clip onto the bike pedals. Eventful tales always followed his group ride experiences when he arrived home, and I remember well that his goal was always to stay in the pack. For non-cyclists, here's a little background. When you ride your bicycle, you are opposing the wind all by yourself, and you exert lots of energy doing so. If you ride with a group of people, the person in front cuts the wind for the group, and the pedaling is much easier and faster for those in the rear. When a large group cycles together, they rotate turns being the lead cyclist so that everyone shares the burden, and everyone benefits from the wind deflection. This group is called a peloton. All cyclists want to stay in the peloton, because getting separated means you're dropped. It's next to impossible to get back in, and a rider will have to cut the wind by himself, the peloton surging ahead and quickly widening the distance. It does not slow down and wait for anyone, and no one lags back to help the dropped rider. Brisk crosswinds, cresting a rise, or being physically out of shape can cause the separation and add to the risk of getting dropped.

If you're in a late stage of your disease, you've probably lost contact with the peloton. You can't do as many things as you once did, and you can't do them as fast. Some days you can't do much at all. Your pace has slowed, and you find that your participation in life is marginal. Perhaps your condition has not yet progressed to that point, but ultimately, it will. Maybe you're a little afraid of this. I know I have had a few mental skirmishes with this, and I doubt if I'm done contending with this unfamiliar way of doing life. As of this writing, I am dealing with this very issue. I do not know how to pace myself very well. I tend to schedule more than I'm able to really accomplish without becoming exhausted. I'm trying to do the things I've been accustomed to doing, but it's hard. It's too early to just withdraw from life. There is a time when we are still involved in it and want to participate, but our participation level has to scale back. To catch up with others is impossible. How to keep moving without comparing your pace with everyone else's is the game.

Moving slowly through a day almost feels forbidden. Like I'm going to get caught and reprimanded. I am not used to doing exactly what I feel like, whenever I feel like it. I have never been one to spend a day at rest and have always enjoyed having a project in the works. Now, if anyone were to observe my day's activities, they would see slothfulness. I do small chores here and there with many rests in between. I do not get up early. Still, I nap in the afternoons. In my sewing room, the light is seldom on, and the tools and art supplies lie dormant. There are so many things I want to do, but my body doesn't feel up to it. Sometimes this is frustrating because I feel as if I am being lazy. I want to go out to lunch with my friends. I wanted to go to Bible study the other day. I want to work on my flower beds. My body says no, you are not up to it. My mind then has two choices: to be angry and frustrated, depressed that I cannot do what I want, or to accept that this is a new plateau. I must find useful things to do that are achievable, but admittedly it's another step down in the decline of my physical body. Accepting it, then, opens a new way of experiencing life in the slow lane.

To do everyday things in slow motion can be an enjoyable meditation if there are no outside pressures or expectations. My day is similar to Angela's. It looks like this: up at around 8:00 a.m., personal maintenance, breakfast, and bed making take up the next two hours, twice the time it once took. Then, I am tired from the exertion and must rest for an hour or so of napping or reading. Then, maybe a chore like laundry or figuring out dinner and gathering ingredients for a bit of prep. Then I'm tired again and need another rest. The whole day goes like this until bedtime. If I meet a friend, I will need an hour or two afterward to rest. Why detail something so mundane? I want anyone who is in a state of decline to recognize that this is what it looks like for everyone else, too. It's tempting to think you're the only one accomplishing so little. You're not. Working and socializing are fun, but it takes more energy than we realize. What's hard about this now is that only a few weeks ago, I could manage a full social schedule, but now, cutting back is essential. It means saying no to some activities and some people. Conserving energy for the time I want to spend with close friends and family is essential and failing to conserve means not being attuned to them because my tank is low, and my attention span is short. It's okay to say no to priority number two items so we can be fully charged for our number one priorities.

One of my heroines is former missionary Elizabeth Elliot, the wife of Jim Elliot who was killed by Aucas in Ecuador only a short time after he and Elizabeth were married and had a child. I have watched countless hours of her speaking on YouTube videos, and I savor her good common sense and wise counsel. Now deceased, she has left an extraordinary legacy in print and in public addresses, as well as the ordinary life she lived with eternity in mind.

When Jim was killed, Elizabeth was, of course, devastated. She did not move back to the states with her small daughter, though, as I think most of us would. Incredibly, she stayed in Ecuador and continued her missionary work, eventually forgiving and befriending Jim's murderers, living among them and having the tremendous blessing of witnessing God's work in their tribe as they changed from a blood vengeance economy to a grace and forgiveness one. Long before these rewarding, miraculous events occurred, though, she had many ordinary days full of toil and grief and frustration. She relates that the only way she could get through each day despite her profound sorrow over Jim's death was to simply, "Do the next thing." She read her Bible, wrote in her journal, continued her mission work, and went about household tasks, doing the next thing, because there was always a next thing to be done.

For each of us, "the next thing" will be different, but we all have a next thing that needs doing.

For each of us, "the next thing" will be different, but we all have a next thing that needs doing. We might do it slowly, but if we can do it, we will complete the day knowing we did what we could to contribute. I say these words to myself often when I do not know what to do to make the best use of my time. "Do the next thing" always leads me to some small thing that needs to be done. A lightbulb changed, a button sewn on, a salad chopped, a thank-you card written. Sometimes it's a nap taken.

Today was a full day for me. I made the bed, took care of personal grooming, watered the plants, corresponded with a few people, washed a load of towels, visited a friend, did some writing, attended a meeting, and will end the day with devotions. For some, this looks like very little. At one time in my life, I could have done all of this in a couple of hours. Life in the slow lane, doing the next thing one thing at a time, includes resting in between. There have been and likely will be days where all that happens is that we wake up and are glad if we can manage to take care of our own grooming. For now, we can be thankful that we are able to do these next things.

Elizabeth's "next thing" was done with focus and deliberation to keep her sane and grounded. Why have we always thought more and faster were better? Now that we are finding our way in our new and down-shifted gear, we can do things more mindfully and meditatively. Folding laundry? Pray for the person whose clothes we are handling. Preparing food? Pray for those who harvested it, sold it, and will eat it. Need to lie down and rest? Go through the alphabet of people you know, praying for each as you come to their letter. Nothing is really mundane at all, if we consider the possibilities. This idea isn't new at all, but perhaps it should be revisited. Our culture doesn't seem to acknowledge this, and even in our churches, I wonder if much is said about the gospel's application in the everyday-ness of choosing our clothes, making our bed, or sweeping the porch, yet for many of us, these small acts comprise our days.

A dear friend gave me the most beautiful books recently. The embossed covers and gold-leaf edges promise much, and the words inside deliver well. They are entitled *Every Moment Holy*, Volume I and *Every Moment Holy*, Volume II.[12] Each identifies every conceivable part of an ordinary day with a liturgy to accompany it. For those in churches that do not use much liturgy, think of a liturgy like this: a routinely used practice to bring attention to the Lord in whatever we are doing. We can do this in worship at church, or we can do this when worshiping alone, as we go about our daily business. In Volume I, we find this example, from "A Liturgy for Domestic Days":

> Many are the things that must be daily done.
> Meet me therefore, O Lord,
> in the doing of the small, repetitive tasks.
>
> In the cleaning and ordering and
> maintenance and stewardship of things—
>   of dishes, of floors, of carpets
>   and toilets and tubs,
>   of scrubbing and sweeping
>   and dusting and laundering—
> That by such stewardship I might bring
> a greater order to my own life,
> and to the lives of any I am given to serve,
> so that in those ordered spaces
> bright things might flourish:
> fellowship and companionship,
> creativity and conversation,
> learning and laughter and
> enjoyment and health.[13]

We have been plucked out of the fast lane, yes. But the slow lane has much to offer. To find that every ordinary moment is holy when we recognize that we live them *coram deo*, before the face of God; this is encouraging for us when we can perform a mere fraction of what we once could. It encourages us because however much, or little, we do, we do it for the glory of God, which gives each moment meaning and purpose. I

Corinthians 10:31 instructs, "So, whether you eat or drink, or whatever you do, do all to the glory of God." In obedience to this, we can consider each of our activities consecrated to Him. In Volume I, there are liturgies for the changing of diapers, for gardening, for competitors, for enjoyment of bonfires, for the ritual of morning coffee, for those who work in wood and stone and clay, for those who feel awkward in social gatherings. For everything imaginable . . . and so, as we plod through our days, our plodding need not be with Eeyore heaviness.

We are who we have always been: made in His image, and now, a slower version of that same self. We do what we can, doing it as best we can, and we can be satisfied that if we did it for His glory, He is satisfied with our effort. Some now housebound were once those with influence and titles. Some busily worked with skillful hands in critical infrastructure. Some spent lives caring for small children, the elderly, or the disabled. Others worked in the arts. Whoever we are now, our once-busy lives have been curtailed, our skill diminishing with disuse. We need not lament those losses. Psalm 131:1-2 comforts the once-bustling but now becalmed:

> O Lord, my heart is not lifted up; my eyes are not raised too high: I do not occupy myself with things too great and too marvelous for me. But I have calmed and quieted my soul, like a weaned child with its mother; like a weaned child is my soul within me

Here is a good place to describe heroes of the faith such as Joni Eareckson Tada, whose life perfectly exemplifies what I am trying to convey. Surely there is no one living who doesn't know her story, but if there be readers who do not, stop what you're doing right now and look her up. Her story of faith in adversity is astonishing. Nevertheless, I will not tell it because I have a story much nearer than Joni's. The one I would like to describe is my mother. She might be irritated to find herself in a chapter entitled "Life in the Slow Lane." She has been anything but slow, and only now that she is in her seventies has her pace slackened (a fraction). She grew up a paraplegic in an era before the Americans With Disabilities Act of 1990 and even before its precursor, the Rehabilitation Act of 1973. These legislative enactments make provisions for those among us with disabilities so that they may access mass transit and public facilities. They are the reason for wheelchair parking spaces, wide doorways, wide public restrooms stalls, lowered drinking fountains and sinks, level entrance and exit points, ramps from curb to curb at crossings, and many other necessities without which the disabled would be relegated to their own homes as they once were.

I have a story much nearer than Joni's. The one I would like to describe is my mother.

Home is exactly where my mother was kept, because there were so many places she could not go. While she has not lived with a terminal illness and has not felt poorly or had low energy, she has been grounded to her own home for long periods of time, depending on others to get her out and about. Until she learned to drive in 1975, her life was primarily a domestic one. Born in 1945 at the height of the polio epidemic, she contracted it at twelve months old. Polio did not affect cognition in its sufferers, only mobility and/or coordination. In Mom's case, she was unable to walk, which meant that public schools, sidewalks, stores, movie theaters, and public restrooms were all off limits to her. Anywhere the average person could expect to go, she could not go without assistance.

I was born in 1964, witness to these conditions and living within them myself because my mother could not drive. From her, I did not learn about the unfairness of it all. I did not learn that we were stuck at home, or that we had nothing to do since we couldn't go anywhere. I did not learn that everyone else was having fun except for us. She could have held that attitude, but I never once heard her say or even imply anything of the sort. Instead, I observed her to make full use of her time, taking full advantage of everything around her to live a creative, fun, and interesting life.

Those hours spent at home with a mother unable to drive meant that I learned to read by age three. She had a small collection of books for me, and I learned that reading and writing and drawing were fun ways to pass the time. I did not have every toy imaginable, but whatever toys I lacked, she would make. I had Barbie dolls, and she made their clothes on her ancient sewing machine. She made their furniture out of things most people would toss in the trash. I learned never to say I was bored and never to say, "There's nothing to do," because those forbidden words quickly earned chores, teaching me that there was plenty to do if I couldn't figure out how to entertain myself. She kept our house spotless, sang along with Aretha Franklin or Al Green on the eight-track while she cleaned, and spent her spare time writing little poems and sketching pictures. She spent plenty of time talking to her friends and family on the wall phone with the long twirly cord, too. We had lots of company for whom she always had something freshly baked along with a pot of coffee ready to go. People came to our house to have their hair done since she had a natural knack for it. She lacked the use of her legs, but the dexterity in her hands more than made up for it.

I learned never to say I was bored and never to say, "There's nothing to do," because those forbidden words quickly earned chores . . .

I learned that while the world zoomed by outdoors and we were marooned at home, we were the ones with the advantage. I learned how to make something out of nothing. I learned that boredom is a state of mind unrelated to one's circumstances. I learned that if there is something we need and we can't hop in the car to go and get it, we can be resourceful and figure out another way to get things done. In short, she taught me to look for possibilities, and to be content whether alone or with others. Whining was never tolerated, and excuse-making was out of the question. She did not engage in these herself, and I certainly would not get by with it. Never an enabler, she gently pushed me toward independence and encouraged me to figure things out for myself, depending on others as little as possible.

I have made my mother sound saintly and brilliant. She was. But she would be quick to point to the source of her strength. It was God. She spent much time in prayer and in reading her Bible, and these sustained her during the long hours at home with an only child, and after I went to school, they were long hours alone in a house far out into the country. She used this time to build up her faith and did not waste it on worldly cares.

In the mid-1970s, Dad helped Mom to drive. He installed hand controls in our red Chevrolet station wagon. Mom drove up and down our long driveway by herself until she got up the courage to drive around the country square mile alone, then repeated it until she felt confident enough for her driver's exam. At last, she earned her driver's license, dramatically increasing her options and her confidence. She got a job and learned the skill of metrology, the building and repair of aircraft instruments. This work was well-suited for her, as she had always been mechanically minded and curious about how things worked.

For many of us, work has a way of interfering with our devotional time, but not Mom. I mentioned in an earlier passage that she read her Bible before work. This meant rising at 4:30 a.m. each morning faithfully. She wheeled her coffee and her Bible to the big bathroom countertop for reading and prayer time in the still morning silence. Her priorities did not waver.

Now that Mom is in her later seventies, Recurrent Polio Syndrome has emerged. It began a few years ago and is a condition few doctors are familiar with. Many who suffered polio years ago are finding that because of damage to nerve endings, a common set of symptoms presents later in life, including muscle aches, fatigue, brain fog, among others. Because she can care for herself and live independently as a retired senior, she can rest as needed and manage her energy. She can anticipate a busy day ahead by planning restful time before and after. She has learned to do projects in small increments. While she is not terminally ill, she does have a condition that has braked her speed and demanded respite. She is undaunted, having learned from long experience how to adapt and overcome. Surely those of us whose speed has been braked by illness can follow her example. We can heed Beth's advice in the first sentence of this chapter, "The word of the day is energy conservation!

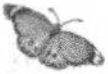

Those who have never learned to be content alone or at home for long periods may struggle with an illness or condition that prevents them from going all the time. Having "nothing to do" can result in hours of TV or phone time. If that is what one chooses, there is no shame. But there is a vast world of choices when we are home, or even home alone for long periods. Within each of us is a reservoir of creativity, and when we are forced to take it slow, we can tap into it and discover things we never knew we might enjoy. I think many discovered this during our COVID-19 isolation. Some despaired while others got creative, and to be fair, those who despaired may have had fewer resources to work with.

One thing we all sought during those long months was to relieve boredom, something I had learned early on out of necessity.

My mother quickly learned that when I was "bored," and she began listing things I could do, I would come back with a whiny response of not wanting to do whatever she was brainstorming. She figured out fast that by making the suggestions for me, she was taking on far too much responsibility for my need to be entertained. Rather, she made it my job to figure out my own recreation, and so I did. Most of the time, my entertainment became something worthwhile—a few chapters read, a stroll outside or some endeavor that didn't require a device or another person. Those who are now mostly housebound are also capable of finding interesting and worthwhile things to do while "stuck," and may even learn to enjoy the time, especially knowing the time is lived before the face of God and for his glory, knowing all we need to do is to "do the next thing."

"The word of the day is energy conservation."

Having plenty of time on our hands can also turn our minds to more spiritual matters as well. What would God have us do? For whom would he have us pray? Who might need a word of encouragement in a text or a card in the mail? On some days, too, even sending a card sounds like a monumental task. Those of us terminally ill are not simply house-bound. Sometimes we are bound within our own bodies. We are wearing down and finding a need for more and more rest. But even this is not cause for discouragement. It is the natural progression and is to be expected. These Scriptures give hope and encouragement:

- Let us remember that Paul, in 2 Corinthians 4:16, tells us not to lose heart! "Though our outer self is wasting away, our inner self is being renewed day by day." Think of that. Our spirit is growing and becoming enriched by His presence even as our earthly husk is withering away! We are preparing for our journey to the afterlife, and we can use this time now to our advantage.

- 2 Corinthians further encourages in 4:17-18: "For this light momentary affliction is preparing for us an eternal weight of glory beyond all comparison, as we look not to the things that are seen but to the things that are unseen, For the things that are seen are transient, but the things that are unseen are eternal." We have begun to flicker out of earthly existence as discussed earlier, and it is a good thing, as we look more and more to our next Home.
- Referring to the human body as a tent, 2 Corinthians 5:1 promises, "For we know that if the tent that is our earthly home is destroyed, we have a building from God, a house not made with hands, eternal in the heavens." We will have a heavenly body, an eternally existing one that far surpasses the one we inhabit now.
- As we spend our time alone, in slow motion, resting and contemplating our lives past, present, and future, we can rest well in the knowledge of 2 Corinthians 3:18: "And we all, with unveiled face, beholding the glory of the Lord, are being transformed into the same image from one degree of glory to another. This comes from the Lord who is the Spirit." As we move into our chrysalis stage, we know we will melt down and transform before we take flight. We need not fear or grieve for long; we can embrace our situation and relax into the knowledge that He is preparing us for metamorphosis.

Life in the slow lane may be one of our last earthly gifts from our Creator. We can finally breathe, not consumed with a long "to do" list. No one is expecting much of us anymore, and we aren't on a dozen committees. It is easy to default to seeing ourselves as victims of our illness, and in a sense, we are, but we need not let ourselves be defined as such. We may be increasingly dependent on others physically, but we can lift others up by our attitudes. We can still exercise compassion and kindness. We can still pray. Let's accept this gift of quiet time with gratitude and ask how God would have us use it for our family's good and for His glory.

Your Reflections

1. What has your experience of being dropped from the peloton been like?

2. What does your typical day look like now that you have downshifted?

3. What simple activities fill your day that you now realize are lived *coram deo*—before the face of God—and how does that knowledge change the way you see these activities?

4. If you were to author a section of *Every Moment Holy*, what liturgies might be included (Example: a liturgy of waxing the car, of changing the sheets, of chopping the salad)?

5. What friends, family, or acquaintances might also be living in the slow lane, and what might you consider doing to companion them?

6. Who are your examples of people who have lived in the slow lane for a long time, and what does their example (or non-example) teach you?

7. If you really wanted to make the worst of your situation right now, what would you do?

8. What might your "do the next thing" practice look like?

9. Who is watching you, and perhaps learning from your example of how to handle a decelerating life?

10. *Prayer:* Write your own prayer, a liturgy of some aspect of ordinary life, that applies to you.

Chapter Eight

Showered Blessings

Finding hidden gifts brings joy and gratitude.

How can we bring closure to our lives in praise and thanksgiving to God?

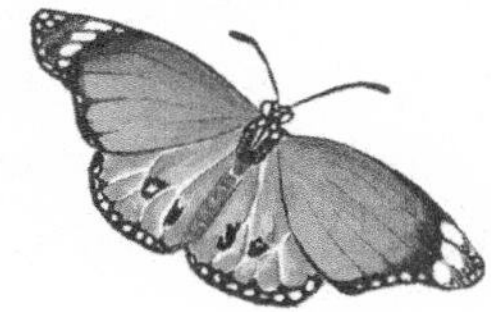

"Listen to your body," medically wise ones advise. Not so easily done when our minds are engaged with external endeavor. My history is one of mind ignoring body. I wouldn't be writing this book or discussing death if I had listened when it was screaming for help a few years ago. The advice is good, because our bodies begin telling us something isn't right long before there's a real problem. Being a slow learner, I've made a discovery of late. Sometimes I am irritable. The slightest word or suggestion provokes an inflammatory reaction where I ruminate on the subject over which I am so irritated, and soon I am feasting on its poison instead of nourishing my spirit with a prayerful attitude and positive thoughts.

The discovery is that when I am in this state of mind, it is usually accompanied by physical pain. Irritation—emotional turmoil—is usually my first clue that my body is in physical pain. Pain doesn't register as pain immediately for me. I just find myself feeling weighed down, grumpy, and set off by absolutely anything. The cat (why can't he leave me alone?), a gust of wind (I hate wind. Why does Kansas have to be so windy?), the fact that it's morning (I hate morning. I need coffee.). The phone rings (If this is a phone solicitor I'm going to let them have it!). I try to keep this ugliness concealed, not wanting to be known as a complaining malcontent. Sadly, God knows, and I doubt I'm as good at hiding it as I think I am.

And then I realize it: I do not feel well. It is time to take my pain meds. Looking at the schedule, I see that I was due for a dose half an hour ago and I had forgotten. Or it's early morning and I allowed myself to sleep without an alarm notification that it's medicine time, which means I am awakened by a foul mood, and then I notice the pain. Even before cancer, this was still true. Pain registered first as a mood shift.

One day in my classroom I was in a thunderous mood, annoyed by my students, co-workers, piles of ungraded papers, emails both read and unread. I knew something wasn't right and I seldom had a day where I disliked my job, but this day I hated it. Students cleared my room after a mid-morning bell and all was quiet as my planning time began, and that's when I noticed how badly my head hurt. So badly that I needed to be picked up and taken home, unable to drive, vomiting as I walked in the door with a massive migraine. Eventually, after hours in the dark, it abated. I was puzzled over how angry I was over nothing just before feeling the migraine. How could I not have realized what was happening? Does this even matter?

Pain registered first as a mood shift.

I think it does. These nasty little ruminations, when taken together, frame an attitude, and once that attitude is set for the day, it is easily maintained by an ordinary comment that I now perceive as provoking.

If those thoughts take root in my mind, I can spend the next thirty minutes mulling over past conversations, nursing slights from the past and dredging up old grievances that I thought were buried. This is a meditation of the wrong kind. It's saturating my mind with toxicity and if I am listening to my body, I notice these kinds of thoughts feel heavy and burdensome. I am only making my initial problem of pain worse.

Along with the discovery that pain is usually the driving force behind my petulance, is the ability to catch myself in the act. A little alarm goes off that tells me to stop, go take my meds, get seated or lie down comfortably, and do something positive until it takes effect, such as reading or journaling. It works. The attitude dissolves as the pain abates. This, too, is a meditation, of the kind that makes us feel better now that we are listening to our bodies. This is no small thing if we value relationships, or if we like feeling joy and lightheartedness. Those things suffer and die if we do not kill the attitude before it grows. I am often alone during the day, so the problem doesn't have a chance to be cast onto others anywhere other than in my mind. But it has happened that I've been caught off guard when with others, and the barbed comment, eye roll, or too-loud sigh has leaked my internal toxicity and caused in hurt feelings. If attitude were insignificant, it would not be mentioned in the Bible, but as it happens, mentions of attitude are found everywhere from Genesis to Revelation, and Scripture reveals that our attitudes are subject to our dictates.

Our thoughts can be trained.

Our thoughts can be trained. Not easy, but possible. Paul gives the instruction to "take every thought captive to obey Christ" (2 Corinthians 10:5b). He is discussing thoughts in a different context here, but the point taken for our purpose is that we can take our thoughts captive. They need not run amok, unrestrained, subjecting us to their imagined tyranny. We can have mastery over them.

Further, Paul concludes his letter to the Philippians about the peace he has in Christ, telling them he has learned to be content in every situation. In 4:8, he advises, "Finally, brothers, whatever is true, whatever is honorable, whatever is just, whatever is pure, whatever is lovely, whatever is commendable, if there is any excellence, if there is anything worthy of praise, think about these things." Again, we can direct our thoughts onto whatever subject matter we select. It isn't enough to tell ourselves to stop being irritable, or to cease negativity. This doesn't work.

Instead, we can capture the ones we don't want and replace them with higher and better ones. From gracious thoughts flow kind and considerate words. We need not use pain as an excuse, either. A bonus discovery was that my thoughts can be captured and changed before medications even take effect, which means that it's all a matter of being aware that my internal state needs to be governed just as much as my external state. For me, pain is the trigger. Once it has been fired, I'm soon thinking about every conceivable depressing thing, worrying about people, fussing over things I can't control. It's good to have knowledge of how to escape this mental prison now, before my condition declines further, and a good meditation is to practice thinking on whatever is good, true, and beautiful.

Perhaps you are triggered by something else. Dwelling on our prognosis can push us down the slide into mental quicksand. Feeling lonely at having been left behind the peloton. Realizing how far you have wandered from God. Lacking a solid inner circle of support. Pondering on loss. Whatever the catalyst is for your own negative thoughts, you'll notice that the negative thinking spirals downward, driving you into a small, mean place in your spirit. Does this mean we aren't allowed to grieve? Is lament never an acceptable frame of mind when circumstances overwhelm us to the point of despair?

It is unfair to underestimate the gravity of what we are handed sometimes. We need to cry, to hurl the ugly words into the journal, to isolate for a while as we let the waves of sadness roll over us. To be crushed by the heartbreak of knowing those we love will be here without us (but if it were not so, we would eventually be here without them). Things that are too terrible for words happen to us or those we know, and it isn't appropriate to be a false fountain of positivity. It's okay that our honest initial reaction is fear or anger or despair. We don't have to pretend everything is fine. We are suffering.

Paul Tripp has written a book sharing his own health crisis and consequently altered life entitled *Suffering: Gospel Hope When Life Doesn't Make Sense.*[14] He knows first-hand that,

> Suffering is never just a matter of the body but is always also a matter of the heart. It's never just an assault on our situation, but also an attack on our soul. Suffering takes us to the borders of our faith.

It is a massive blow that is not easily absorbed, and Tripp explains that we may get caught up focusing on the physical nature of suffering, forgetting that our mind and spirit suffer as well. Spiritual warfare is at work here and our enemy is always eager to help us suffer in ways that cause us to question faith, lament unfairness, and bring us to despair.

The good news is that we aren't stuck there and don't have to stay. Besides knowing we can capture our thoughts and redirect them, it is also good to remember that our trials may also be a test of faith.

> . . . so that the tested genuineness of your faith—more precious than gold that perishes though it is tested by fire—may be found to result in praise and glory and honor at the revelation of Jesus Christ. (1 Peter 1:7)

Even amid such trials, we have assurance that: "The Lord is near to all who call on him . . . " (Psalm 145:18). Many, including myself, know this is true, having lived it. Those who have experienced this supernatural peace while suffering also know that the only response is mind-blowing, overwhelming gratitude.

When you learned of your diagnosis, was gratitude the first thing that came to mind? It takes a while for our new status to settle. We need a minute to figure out what our new health status is going to mean, how it's going to redefine our lives. When the sediment of our disturbance has had time to settle, to work its way into our center, unexpected stirrings may begin a transformation in us that we could not have expected.

Thanksgiving is a powerfully transformative mindset to hold and principle to guide us.

Once our tears ducts have been depleted and our fight has been spent (or better yet, we recognize there never was a fight to begin with), we can do an astonishing thing: we can look back in a review of our lives and be thankful. We can also look at our surroundings and be thankful. We can even give thanks for the condition we've been resisting, not because we like it, but because of the innumerable good things that have come of it.

Thanksgiving is a powerfully transformative mindset to hold and principle to guide us, as we are repeatedly instructed in Scripture, ". . . give thanks in all circumstances; for this is the will of God in Christ Jesus for you" (1 Thessalonians 5:18). Yes, in all circumstances. Psalm 28:7 praises, "The Lord is my strength and my shield; in him my heart trusts, and I am helped; my heart exults, and with my song I give thanks to him." Numerous Psalms contain similar thanks and praise passages. Gratitude echoes throughout the pages of Scripture from beginning to end, so it is right for us to take our cues from it and discover its power.

It is noteworthy that Jesus gave thanks frequently. Here, before sharing the bread and wine at the Last Supper:

> Now as they were eating, Jesus took bread, and after blessing it broke it and gave it to the disciples, and said, "Take, eat; this is my body." And he took a cup, and when he had given thanks he gave it to them, saying, "Drink of it, all of you, for this is my blood of the covenant, which is poured out for many for the forgiveness of sins." (Matthew 26:26-27)

When we celebrate the body and blood of Christ in the Eucharist, we are giving thanks for the very elements that secured our salvation. We are reminded of His body, broken for us. His blood, spilled for us, as atonement for our sin.

At one time I thought of sin as a series of bad behaviors that I needed to overcome before I could truthfully call myself a Christian. This is not at all what the gospel is about. If we could eradicate bad behaviors and get our lives together on our own, Jesus' work on the cross was in vain. Sin is not a series of bad behaviors. It is a condition into which we are born as offspring of our first parents, Adam and Eve, whose fall set the pattern for mankind.

Sin puts self in the center. It manifests in a variety of outward behaviors, but ultimately, it is a "self above others" condition. Sin looks different on each of us, as the particular sins for which we have a propensity come to light. Formerly invisible to us, allowing us to think we are basically good people, the light of His holiness allows us a glimpse into our true condition. Once we see in the mirror that Christ holds up for us, we are moved to repentance, seeking His forgiveness and grace, which is freely given. With gratitude, we begin to understand what God has done for us: He has given His son to pay the penalty due to us by dying the painful, humiliating death of crucifixion. And then, His shocking resurrection on the third day crushes the horror of death once and for all. These passages give further assurance of our eternal home:

- 2 Corinthians 5:8 softens the fear of death, saying, "Yes, we are of good courage, and we would rather be away from the body and at home with the Lord."
- 1 Corinthians 15:55 accomplishes the same: "O death, where is your victory? O death, where is your sting?" We have nothing to fear in death if we are in Christ."
- 1 Peter 1:3 alludes to a glorious eternity, proclaiming "Blessed be the God and Father of our Lord Jesus Christ! According to his great mercy, he has caused us to be born again to a living hope through the resurrection of Jesus Christ from the dead . . . "

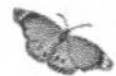

At home. My father-in-law spoke this truth a few days before his physical death. He knew that to be with the Lord was to truly be home. We know what home is, or what we wish it were. It is not only a place we eat, sleep and store our temporal treasures. It is a place where we feel secure and able to rest. It is a sanctuary we create that is filled with things we enjoy; a place we share with those we love, offering hospitality. We like to keep our homes peaceful, a refuge from the world and a shelter from the elements. We find most of these elements and more in our promise of a Heavenly home, first referenced in chapter four, and re-emphasized here as we consider what it means to go home. Jesus says in John 14:2: "In my Father's house are many rooms. If it were not so, would I have told you that I go to prepare a place for you?" This gift of eternal life, dwelling with Him eternally, is the ultimate gift for which we owe Him boundless gratitude. We long to go to our earthly home at the end of a long trip away, but as our earthly lives expire, we increasingly long for the home He has prepared for us.

Gratitude is a habit, a practice, a meditation, a proactive effort that must be taken on with intention but fueled by the Spirit that indwells us. In the Gospel of Matthew, we find in 5:16, " . . . let your light shine before others, so that they may see your good works and give glory to your Father who is in heaven." Grumbling and complaining tend to dull this light that we are exhorted to shine, but hearts full of gratitude spill that light into the darkest corners. When we ask the Holy Spirit to show us these gifts—what God has done for us, what He has made, the intricacy of creation, the glory of His plans—we cannot help but overflow with thanksgiving as they are revealed.

When we look back over our lives, perhaps we can see in our little microcosm how, over time, God has had His hand on us, guiding us the entire time. At the time, we didn't know what God was doing. We didn't know how our choices would lead to future consequences, good or bad. Now that we have come to the end, we see that life cannot be fully understood in the present; it is only in retrospect that it all begins to make sense. Danish theologian Soren Kierkegaard expressed it with eloquent brevity: "Life can only be understood backwards, but it must be lived forward."

Because we do not know what lies ahead, subject as we are to living in the moment, it is easy to succumb to anxiety. Philippians 4:6 instructs, "Do not be anxious about anything, but in everything by prayer and supplication with thanksgiving let your requests be made known to God." In everything . . . with thanksgiving. Not just when it's all going your way, but in everything, because he knows the outcome, and it will ultimately be for our good and His glory. Trust, look for the gifts and see His provision.

To do this, Ann Voskamp tells us in her book, *One Thousand Gifts: A Dare to Live Fully Right Where You Are*, we must slow down.[15] Then it's a good thing we are living in the slow lane. Here's something achievable for us. We're no longer in the peloton, racing to stay abreast of the others, after all. She directs the reader to Psalm 39:6, "Surely a man goes about as a shadow! Surely for nothing they are in turmoil . . . " We do a lot of rushing around, and much of it comes to nothing. Voskamp continues, "In our rushing, bulls in china shops, we break our own lives." And then, the pulse of her thesis strikes us, those who have spent life being busy, thinking we have too little time:

> I . . . realize for the first time what has never been the problem of my life. The real problem of life is never a lack of time. The real problem of life—my life—is lack of thanksgiving.

I wish I had known this as a young mother. That "life is not an emergency," as Voskamp puts it." It is *eucharisteo* . . . that in Christ, what is most urgent necessitates a slow and steady reverence."

How could we notice the gifts if we are multitasking through every day? If everything is a flaming emergency, we are unable to find the time to give thanks. To slow down for us is now easy. And now, it is a delight for us to find the gems hidden everywhere. Small ones and huge ones. She keeps a notebook on her nightstand, by her kitchen sink, in her purse, seeking to capture each one, not letting anything escape her notice. If she, a homeschooling mother of six (now seven) can do this as well as write books, we have no excuse not to notice the good that abounds. To see and think on what is true, honorable, just, pure, lovely, commendable, excellent, and praiseworthy.

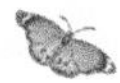

My friend Ann is not terminal. She didn't know that, though, when she had the COVID-19 Delta variant forcefully attack her lungs shortly after a week of what just seemed like a weird cold. With her nursing background, she had faith in her medical knowledge and was comfortable following the advised Covid protocols, trusting that she would recover easily. On day seven, she found out otherwise. With oxygen saturation levels plummeting to 77%, she began to panic, all faith in her medical expertise gone. By a series of divinely orchestrated events, she quickly had medicine on her doorstep that reversed the growing catastrophe in her lungs, which cleared within an hour. This was day seven, and the Covid roller coaster she was on would take months to stop. Her prayers in days before the frantic gasping for oxygen had begun were that God's will be done, whatever that might mean. Because of His indwelling Spirit, she was able to recognize that either way, she would be in good hands. The result was "peace and an odd contentment" even as her body panicked for oxygen; her spirit was serene, experiencing the presence of God. Because of the perfect timing of the delivered medicine, her lungs cleared and filled with oxygen once again, but Covid was far from finished with her.

How could we notice the gifts if we are multitasking through every day?

Ann's fever spiked and her oxygen saturation dropped again, but at that moment, her doctor called her. Whose doctor does that? This was not typical for her doctor either, but again, the timing was perfect, and soon, two other medications were on board that once again reversed the decline. Friends and family surrounded her, providing meals, bringing oxygen, and praying. The days melted together as she slept off and on, others caring for every need. She knew that God arranged it all, and with impeccable timing. As it seemed things were improving, another setback occurred.

She was out of a needed medication and was again declining but was shown what to do to hang on until it arrived a few days later. Her brain was hypoxic, her thinking clouded much of the time, but she had pure clarity at critical moments, knowing what to do to prevent further decline—information that she knows did not originate in her own mind. Her initial anxiety at being out of medicine calmed as she took it captive, trusting in God's continued care regardless of the circumstance. She also remembered her prayer that His will be done. Once again, she was enjoying His presence, knowing that in Him we live, and move, and have our being, praying often through Ephesians. She relates, "Every breath we take is a gift from Him, who is our Life and Light and Presence!" The medicine eventually did arrive, and Ann seemed to be improving.

Covid then attacked her circulation and aggravated her Reynaud's Syndrome, sending her into a another steep decline. A friend had left a particular drug with her "just in case" she might need it, then texted her to urge her to take it. Reluctantly, she finally did and got instant, unexpected relief. Over and over, provision just in time, so obviously not the work of humans, but of God's work through them. Several weeks in, though, she still had no strength. It would take months for the recovery to be complete, and even now, she must manage her energy carefully.

During her illness, she was sustained by God's presence, treasuring intimate knowledge of Him, who was closer to her than any human had ever been. Many sleepless nights were times she cherished as she listened to the audio Bible, knowing His presence and filled with such overwhelming joy that was only possible because of His presence in hardship. Over the winter months, she gradually grew stronger, both grateful for the healing and regretful that as she healed, her sense of His nearness waned.

Now that she is well again, Ann misses being sick. Not the awfulness of Covid itself, but the long period of time during which God's presence sustained her. She wanted to live, but to a greater extent she wanted His will to be done, knowing that " . . . to live is Christ, and to die is gain" (Philippians 1:21). She is now back among the living. God's will was for her healing, and while she is thankful to be alive, the greatest blessings for her were the times spent in His glorious presence.

Ann looks back to this time with awe at God's love, His kindness, and the unity of those he brought together to care for her. She remembers not the physical discomfort or anxiety, but the blessings that came as a result of Covid, many of which are not detailed here. Overflowing with gratitude, she was awe-struck by God's provision of what she needed before she ever prayed for it, astonished by the sweet surprises that He gave her along the way. Ann's trust, immersion in Scripture, prayer, and total surrender that His will be done are instructive for us. She could easily have died at several points but was spared for reasons she does not know. Even though it appears our outcome will be different, her story is edifying, and we can take our cues from her approach to sickness. We, too, can give thanks and look for the blessings.

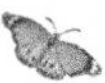

Giving thanks in every circumstance whether it is Covid, cancer, ALS, or any other fatal condition shows our faith in God's goodness and our trust in His sovereignty. He keeps us safe in His care whether He preserves earthly life a bit longer, as with Ann, or brings us home to eternal life, as with you and me. Either way, "Precious in the sight of the Lord is the death of His saints" (Psalm 115:16). Gratitude in every circumstance proclaims that we know He will work everything out for our good and His glory. We trust, even when we do not know how or when He will accomplish His ends.

Giving thanks also purifies our cluttered thoughts. Many of the Psalms begin as bitter complaint and frustration, but end in praise and thanksgiving. When we write our prayers, we may discover the same. My written prayers usually start out messy. Again, my frantic torrent of words slows as the pent-up energy dissipates onto the page, giving way to the sparkling calm that is thanks and praise, cathartic for me, and due to Him. He shows me what He has done for me and mine. I remember that He is good and that His ways are higher than my ways. It is very unlike worrying and pleading for the miracle we desire, assuming we know best. We have no idea what is best, but we can give thanks for what is. We can praise Him for His trustworthiness. We can express faith that He will act in the best way and in the best timing. We can look around and see what is true, honorable, just, pure, lovely, commendable, excellent, and praiseworthy in the meantime, trustfully waiting.

We trust, even when we do not know how or when He will accomplish His ends.

When I first read Voskamp's book several years ago, I was in good health. I enjoyed the book, and I took my cues from her gratitude list suggestions. They were surprisingly simple. For example, gifts that are blue or yellow, rough or smooth—these seemed almost silly at the start, but I found that I enjoyed pondering those simple categories. Making the gratitude lists daily, weekly, and monthly was engaging. I don't know when the practice stopped. I may have skipped a couple of days, allowed myself to do it mentally rather than written, who knows. I remembered the importance of seeking the gifts, but in my current state, I believe it to be even more important.

I have begun the practice again. Resurrecting childhood memories of my mother, I recall that it was in her nature to do this. Having been a city girl moved to the country, she was in awe of newborn calves, steam rising off their wet little bovine bodies in the morning sunlight. She loved the open space and the sounds of life without airplanes and cars and trains. I did too, though I reveled more in the perennial flowers and plants that grew on the grounds of the rented farmhouse. To even continue in this chapter, and to compile my gratitude lists, I needed to do some of the work outdoors. It is easier to write about gratitude when surrounded by singing birds and breezes, soft grass and delicately veined leaves. Now, my lists are just as simple as the ones she suggested. I stop and think back over the past couple of days.

Today's haul: the evening sun's slant across green grass, cottonwood seeds gleaming silver in the sunlight, call of a bird I have not heard before, sound of the garage door when my husband arrived home, sound of a grandson's clear and sweet voice at his choir concert, kind-hearted effort of my granddaughter's compliment on my newly shorn post-chemo hairstyle, another grandson telling us about his bedtime prayers, delight in the life cycle of a butterfly shared by another grandson (we ordered a kit together so that we could observe the stages), juiced carrots, the way the plants perked up after their banana water drink, the ability to clean up the front porch (and live there during summer), my daughter's chicken and garden keeping, my son's thoughtful lyrics, geese, yellow irises blooming by the fence, succulents Eric wintered under a grow light that now populate the outdoors.

These are small details that fuel my joy. It is true that all we have is today, and today has been good. I give thanks for where I have been, where I am, and where I am going, for who I have in this life and those with whom I'll be reunited in the next. And a final thanks is due to the One whose grace makes that possible. For His mercy on me, a sinner in need of grace and for His continued attention to every small detail that, when accrued, has coalesced into this life over which He has presided, provided, and sustained, part of which I have told in these chapters. As it winds down, I trust that as I cross the river to the celestial city, He will sustain my faith so that the passage will be easily crossed, just as it was for Faithful and Christian in *Pilgrim's Progress*, one of my favorite books and a must-read for every Christian.

May your final days be full of gratitude, faith, and hope.

I hope that you, my reader, will find the gifts that surround you, too. May your final days be ones that are full of gratitude, faith, and hope. "Now faith is the assurance of things hoped for, the conviction of things not seen" (Hebrews 11:1). Because we belong together in unity with Him, we will await the

> . . . glorious day of His appearing. But our citizenship is in Heaven, and from it we await a Savior, the Lord Jesus Christ, who will transform our lowly body to be like his glorious body, by the power that enables him even to subject all things to himself. (Philippians 3:20-21)

And then we will truly be home.

> One thing have I asked of the LORD, that will I seek after:
> that I may dwell in the house of the LORD all the days of my life,
> to gaze upon the beauty of the LORD and to inquire in his temple. (Psalm 27:4)

To Myself: A Few Reminders

When days are cut short of the run you'd envisioned
and plans that you made have all perished,

remember the travels and seasons enjoyed,
the colleagues and confidantes cherished.

Do not waste a moment bemoaning your lot,
lamenting your truncated years!

As long as you can, you must do the next thing,
to resist the dark specter of fears.

The sunrise will daily deliver your work,
and you'll joyfully finish each task.

Good cheer will be proffered, companions will ring
and in their rapport you will bask.

No bucket list promise can rival their worth,
neither beaches nor mountainous places.

No rivals can quell your delight in their voices,
nor sight of their four little faces.

Whatever remains of your stay upon earth,
let each of the hours declare

that you're brimming with thanks for the blessings bestowed!
(He has lavished much more than your share)

For home, friends, and family—such plentiful wealth
His generous hand did accord.

To your very last breath let your praises resound
"Alleluia! Christ Jesus is Lord!"

Your Reflections

1. What are some things that trigger negativity for you?

2. What is an example of a time when you found yourself in an emotional mess after being triggered?

3. In what ways do you respond when a foul mood threatens to control you?

4. What toxic thoughts have you caught yourself wallowing in, and what was the result?

5. To what extent have you practiced gratitude (E.g. counting your blessings, looking for gifts)?

6. How comfortable are you with releasing your life to God's will, as Ann did?

7. What does "home" mean to you?

8. Kierkegaard's words, "Life can only be understood backwards, but it must be lived forward," mean that we understand our lives much better when we look back, but we don't know what's going on in the moment. Looking back what evidence do you see that God has had his hand on your entire life?

9. Identify ten small gifts for which you can be thankful today.

10. Give thanks to God in prayer for what He has done in your life, and ask Him to show you the blessings that have come of your illness.

Afterword

An Interview With My Hospice Team

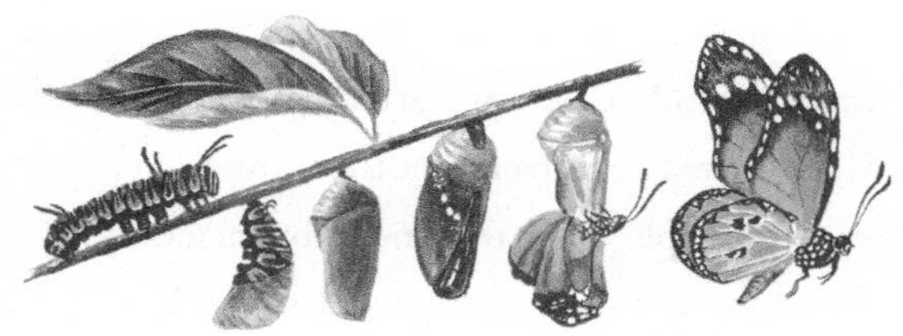

Their remarks are incorporated throughout the chapters, but they made so many interesting comments that I wanted to create a separate section just for their insights. God has gifted Tom, Casie, and Beth, and commissioned them to work with patients and families during the hardest time in their lives, and their wisdom is yet another gift for us.

Do you often encounter people who do not have a support system of friends and family?

Beth: Yes, friend/companion is more the role we play. We facilitate conversations to help people find peace and closure. Lots of time is needed to help build family support or introduce faith and spiritual support.

Casie: Yes. In some instances, we are all they have. I have had patients I visited every day who have no one else. There was one girl in particular who stands out in my mind. She was in her early twenties. One parent was deceased, and the other parent was not in her life. She had no other relatives to companion her. In other cases, I try to facilitate broken relationships as much as I can. Sometimes just pulling in extra resources helps. Having all the necessary support pieces in place sometimes brings the people together. I know of one instance where there was a man who had no one, and by arranging Meals on Wheels, His Helping Hands (for furniture provision), and a few others, a son started getting involved, and is now his full-time caregiver. Another thing I try to remember is to give people what they need by enacting it. For example, if they need to have patience, I try to be very patient with them. If they need love, I try to show love to them. Anger is a secondary emotion, and we have to look past that to see what it is they really need.

Tom: Philippians 2:1-11 speaks of Jesus' suffering while putting others first. Do we really take on caring for the interest of others? One example of this is when I was a chaplain in the ER, and there was a woman who was sitting in the floor, distraught and wailing. The best thing for me to do right then was to meet her where she was at, so I sat on the floor with her. I told her I didn't blame her and I would feel the same way if I were her. It took a while, but she calmed down. We don't try to tell people what to do. We help them figure out what to do. Sometimes it happens that people become more selfless in their last days. They can't do anything else. They will start thinking of what they want to give to others or begin saying things to others that they hadn't before. Sometimes people draw closer to Christ in the end. Family members sometimes do this, too, displaying the humility shown in these verses. Being selfless is something everyone can do, even in their last days.

> So if there is any encouragement in Christ, any comfort from love, any participation in the Spirit, any affection and sympathy, complete my joy by being of the same mind, having the same love, being in full accord and of one mind.
>
> Do nothing from selfish ambition or conceit, but in humility count others more significant than yourselves. Let each of you look not only to his own interests, but also to the interests of others. Have this mind among yourselves, which is yours in Christ Jesus, who, though he was in the form of God, did not count equality with God a thing to be grasped, but emptied himself, by taking the form of a servant,[c] being born in the likeness of men. And being found in human form, he humbled himself by becoming obedient to the point of death, even death on a cross.
>
> Therefore God has highly exalted him and bestowed on him the name that is above every name, so that at the name of Jesus every knee should bow, in heaven and on earth and under the earth, and every tongue confess that Jesus Christ is Lord, to the glory of God the Father (Philippians 2:1-11).

What are your thoughts on why the Bible brings peace to the reader, even more when the reader has a keener sense of mortality?

Tom: The word of God is living and active and fulfills whatever need we have. It is NOT self-help, but God know what we need.

Casie: We are part flesh man, part spirit man. Spirit man is fulfilled when reading God's word. God is the author of peace, not of confusion. Isaiah 40:31 says, " . . . but they who wait for the LORD shall renew their strength; they shall mount up with wings like eagles." We can soar above the storm.

Beth: He is blessing with grace because we are seeking Him. He is always seeking us, so when the seeking is reciprocal, he grants peace.

To encourage those facing their final hours, share with us your experience of seeing people pass in peace?

Casie: This happens when they have confidence in their destination. Those surrounding them can feel that they are at peace.

Tom: People are at peace when they have the hope of Heaven—they have been saved, but are also being saved. The spirit of harmony in the place is discernible, People sometimes sit up in bed, their eyes go bright, they might reach up, or have big smiles.

Beth: Sometimes a peaceful death is an uneventful death, where the patient dies peacefully with no fighting. They often have a peaceful expression. One thing to note: family should not call hospice the moment death occurs but wait at least fifteen minutes or so. Those moments after someone dies are not a time to rush, but to just sit with for a bit. There is something holy about that time. If you are blessed enough to be present when the patient passes, there is a sense of peace and holiness afterward.

What is rewarding/frustrating about your job?

Tom: I want to serve people during difficult times with peace and dignity. Isaiah 57:1-2 is an example where God takes people and it ends up protecting them from something else if they had lived. God knows the other side. Sometimes people want one more year, but there is always one more, and one more. It's also rewarding to be present to non-believers who begin to question their agnostic or atheistic views, and I can share the gospel with them at a time when they're paying attention.

Casie: I want to be part of the picture; part of the peace, honored to be part of people's journey. Patients and families who do not choose the Lord can be frustrating because I have seen that bereavement is harder. In working with families, if there is no harmony, then we try to facilitate it. These are hard conversations.

Beth: I like helping people, getting to know families, and building bonds. When they die, the bond is broken, and that's hard. There is no time to grieve the loss since I need to move on to the next patient. The actual death is hard for me—it is emotionally exhausting. I go home and take a shower, then I need to isolate for a while to let things settle.

What insights might you share regarding our physical care when we are unable to manage it in the last days?

Tom: The idea of "the last bath" is a gift some caregivers have. It is their gifting from God to care for those who are dying and helpless, and it is something they want to do. It is their way of serving the Lord.

Casie: The last bath is another measure to provide relaxation. Getting comfortable is a big deal at the end, and it is an important role for the caregivers who do this.

Beth: Sometimes a person passes when they are turned during their last bath. They become so relaxed that it helps them to let go and pass.

Having been present in situations where hospice has been called in with months to go, or with only days or hours, is there an ideal time to involve hospice care?

Casie and Tom: Hospice is better earlier rather than later—we can get to know families and patients, and we can better serve because it is a longer relationship.

Tom: Our job is to help families discover what to do, not to tell them what to do.

Beth: The earlier the better so I can build a rapport with the patient and family to be a better support for them. I have never heard people say they wish they had waited. I have heard people say they wish they had known and asked earlier for help.

Acknowledgements

So many people have encouraged me to write over the years, and being the procrastinator that I am, I waited until the literal last minutes in my life to do it. But I never believed I had anything worthwhile to say, and I owe gratitude to those who coaxed something out of me, helping to shape it into something cohesive.

With bottomless gratitude, I give thanks for these:

Anne Tjaden, for kick-starting my thoughts about writing this book, offering her encouragement and editing skills.

Jennifer Johnson, for closely reading each chapter and providing scriptural support and thoughtful feedback and encouragement over and over and over.

Amy Edwards, for immensely helpful coaching on an especially challenging section.

Amy Edwards and Tina Mugglin of Blue Sky Daisies, for seeing a need and (shockingly) offering an avenue for publication.

Casie Cooper, Beth Rohling, and Tom Scott, my wonderful hospice team, surely appointed by God for this work.

My mom, Linda Smith and my late father, Pat Smith, for providing much of the inspiration for the content and always being supportive.

Logan and Jill, Jake and Erica, Lincoln, Violet, Gage, and Montana, my treasured people.

Mr. Eric Mize, my husband and president of my inner circle, for wholeheartedly supporting my efforts from the beginning, vowing to get my work published if he had to do it himself, if necessary.

Father, Son, and Holy Spirit, the Source and Recipient of my unending gratitude, my all in all.

Endnotes

1. Vicki A. Jackson, MD MPH; David P. Ryan, MD, *Living With Cancer: A Step-by-Step Guide for Coping Medically and Emotionally With a Serious Diagnosis* (Baltimore: Johns Hopkins University Press, 2017), 273.
2. Sarah Young, *Jesus Calling* (Nashville: Thomas Nelson, 2019).
3. William Bridges, *Managing Transitions: Making the Most of Change* (Cambridge, MA: DeCapo Press, 2003).
4. Ibid.
5. Ibid.
6. Randy Alcorn, *Heaven: A Comprehensive Guide to Everything the Bible Says About Our Eternal Home* (Wheaton, IL: Tyndale House, 2004).
7. John Sammis, *Trust and Obey,* https://library.timelesstruths.org/music/Trust_and_Obey/.
8. Clarence L. Haynes, Jr., "Why 'God Helps Those Who Help Themselves' Is Presumed to Be Biblical," Christianity Today.com, July 7, 2020. https://www.christianity.com/wiki/christian-life/why-god-helps-those-who-help-themselves-is-presumed-to-be-biblical.html.
9. Kurt Vonnegut, *Cat's Cradle* (New York: Dell, 1984).
10. Ira Bock, MD, *The Four Things That Matter Most* (New York: Atria Books, 2004).
11. DermaWand.com.
12. Douglas Kaine McKelvey, *Every Moment Holy,* Vol. 1 (Nashville: Rabbit Room Press, 2017).
13. Ibid, 15.
14. Paul David Tripp. *Suffering: Gospel Hope When Life Doesn't Make Sense* (Wheaton, Illinois: Crossway, 2018), 46.
15. Ann Voskamp, *One Thousand Gifts: A Dare to Live Fully Right Where You Are* (Grand Rapids, MI: Zondervan, 2010).

About the Author

Kelly Mize is wife to Eric Mize, mother of their two grown humans, grandmother of four, former teacher, and cat mom to Mocha. Her written record is found only in yellowed journals, a few scholarly papers, two master's theses, thousands of marginalia remarks on her students' writing, and this first and last book. She and Eric live in Clearwater, Kansas and make Evangel Presbyterian Church, PCA their church home.